Teenage Pregnancy

The Interaction of Psyche and Culture

Teenage Pregnancy

The Interaction of Psyche and Culture

ANNE L. DEAN

in collaboration with

SARAH J. DUCEY
MARY M. MALIK

THE ANALYTIC PRESS

1997   Hillsdale, NJ   London

Akymao

Published by
The Analytic Press, Inc.
Editorial Offices:
101 West Street
Hillsdale, New Jersey 07642

Library of Congress Cataloging-in-Publication Data

Dean, Anne L.
Teenage pregnancy : the interaction of psyche and culture / Anne L. Dean
in collaboration with Sarah J. Ducey, Mary M. Malik.
p.   cm.
Includes bibliographical references and index.
ISBN 0-88163-254-6
1. African American teenage mothers—Louisiana, Southern—Social
conditions.   2. African American teenage mothers—Louisiana, Southern—
Psychology.   3. Unmarried mothers—Louisiana, Southern—Social
conditions.   4. Unmarried mothers—Louisiana, Southern—Psychology.
5. Rural poor—Louisiana, Southern—Social conditions.   6. Rural poor—
Louisiana, Southern—Psychology.   7. Teenage pregnancy—Louisiana,
Southern.   8. Mothers and daughters—Louisiana, Southern.   I. Ducey,
Sarah J.   II. Malik, Mary M.   III. Title.
HQ759.4.D45   1997
306.874'3—dc21   97-29816
                                                                          CIP

Printed in the United States of America

10   9   8   7   6   5   4   3   2   1

Contents

Preface

This book is about pregnancies among unwed, poor, African American teenagers living in the rural River Parish region of southern Louisiana, a corridor of land extending about 100 miles up and down the banks of the Mississippi River. The story told here begins where many others leave off, with a look into the lives and minds of girls and women who are all poor and all come from families who have lived in conditions of poverty, under-employment, racial oppression, discrimination, and restricted educational opportunities in this region for many years. In this population at high risk for teenage pregnancy, many women have become pregnant as teenagers, but many others have not. The primary question asked in the following pages is, how can we account for these different outcomes?

The reason for asking this question is not just to understand more about teenage pregnancy, although that is an important goal in itself. It is also to understand more about culture and psychology and how these two realms of human existence come together in motivating people to action. The general questions asked in this book are, why do people in a given population put so much effort into doing certain things and not others, are individual psychological and cultural constructs truly separable, and are both necessary to explain why people do what they do? If they are, how can we understand the nature of their joint participation in socially significant action patterns?

There are two aspects of this research that are likely to be controversial. One is that I have taken a psychoanalytic–developmental perspective in trying to understand the collective and individual reasons why some girls do and some girls do not become pregnant as unwed teenagers. The questions I asked, the places that I looked for answers, the methods I used to find them, and the conclusions I reached all reflect that perspective. Judith Musick (1993), whose writings about young, poor, and pregnant girls I quote in the first chapter of this book, spoke to some reasons why attention to psychological–developmental issues tends to generate special concern when it is applied to the poor. On the one hand, such a focus appears to unnecessarily complicate a picture that seems understandable on the basis of social, economic, and political factors. On the other hand, it seems to resemble the now discredited "culture of poverty" perspective or "blame-the-victim" viewpoint in which problems are identified as "psychological" simply because people are poor. Whereas I agree with Musick that these are concerns raised by attention to psychological–developmental issues, I do not believe, as I discuss further in this preface and in the book itself, that these issues are unnecessarily complicating or that attention to them is tantamount to blaming the victim.

A second concern is that I, as a White middle-class woman, would attempt to understand the lives and minds of poor African Americans. What does it mean that I would choose to study a population of poor African Americans when adolescent pregnancy is prevalent in the poor White population as well? Can a person who is neither poor nor African American understand what the people in this population think and feel? These questions carry with them the underlying worry that by including only poor African Americans in this study, I divert attention away from the responsibilities of other groups in perpetuating the adolescent pregnancy behavior pattern. In addition, although I purport to understand, perhaps I really cannot, yet still my voice will be heard and acted upon by policymakers to the possible detriment of poor African American families.

These worries are legitimate. If this work is interpreted by those in policy-making positions to mean that teenage pregnancy is exclusively a problem of poor African Americans who are becoming pregnant as unwed teenagers for reasons that have little to do with the social, economic, and political environments in which they live, then two things will be true. First, I will have been misunderstood. Second, the danger might arise that policymakers either will throw up their hands in the belief that nothing can be done or, even worse, might implement punitive policies with regard to poor African Americans. To avoid potential misunderstanding, then, in the remainder of this preface I summarize the work, its focus, methods, and findings, and I attempt to clarify what I do mean by stating frankly what I do not mean.

What the Book Is About

One belief consistent with the psychoanalytic–developmental perspective is that the ultimate reasons why people do things and behave in a certain way are known only to them, and then often only at an unconscious level.

Another belief is that people's reasons for doing things have multiple sources—some stemming from the needs, desires, and goals of the social and cultural groups with which they identify and others from more individual needs, desires, and goals. A third related belief is that all behavior, whether it occurs frequently or infrequently within a society, serves several, often conflicting, purposes simultaneously.

In accordance with these views, my primary focus in this research was on the cultural and individual psychological meanings that teenage pregnancies have for people in this population. In particular, I examined what these meanings are, both conscious and unconscious; the historical, family, and interpersonal contexts in which meanings have developed and are perpetuated over generations; and the relation of meanings to adolescent pregnancy outcomes for two generations of women. I looked for answers to these questions in patterns of people's behavior and verbal discourse, which, more so than explicit statements of belief, can reveal meanings that are hidden from conscious awareness. Similar patterns were identified in two phases of the study using different methodologies with different samples, thus attesting to their validity.

In the first phase of the study, I spent 1 or 2 days a week over a 3-year period visiting a small number of families in and around one town in the River Parish region. In the 1st year, I went with Henry, a graduate student in special education, who helped me tutor children whose parents thought they needed help. When Henry moved on, my 11-year-old daughter accompanied me on many visits to the community, which helped to identify me as a mother with at least that in common with most of the women I came to know. Although I stopped making regular visits after 3 years, I have returned to the community from time to time since then for updates about new developments in people's lives. The material that I gathered in this phase consisted of notes written after the fact summarizing impromptu conversations with men, women, and children; observations of their conversations, interactions and activities; and tape recordings (with permission) of planned, informal interviews with people in which I shared my conjectures and observations and asked for their input. Patterns in people's behavior and thoughts were identified in this material through qualitative analyses.

In contrast to some other studies in which researchers have lived in the communities they studied (e.g., Dougherty, 1978; Ladner, 1971; Stack, 1974), I was not a part of everyday life in this community. Things happened while I was there that I observed and in which I occasionally participated, but I was always clearly an observer looking in from the outside. Still, the methodology I used had the great advantage of time. When I was there, people tolerated and even welcomed my presence when there was no reason not to. They were generally willing to talk to me about themselves, their experiences, plans, hopes, fears, disappointments, and successes—to tell me stories, rumors, and gossip. They invited me to go places with them, asked me to give them rides in my car, offered me food and drink, and were otherwise polite and friendly. I went to county fairs, grocery stores, hospitals, jails, courthouses, and churches with people in the community. With time, I heard and observed many different versions of the same stories, perspectives on the same subject, variations on the same themes, thoughts and feelings of the same people. With time, people stopped telling me what they thought I wanted to hear or what they wanted me to think and started telling me what they did think. In the end, I had a picture of this community that was very different from the one I had in the beginning.

The second phase of the study, which also lasted 3 years, used a very different methodology that complemented the first. Rather than attempting to know a lot about the inner and outer lives of a few people, we determined to know enough about the thoughts, feelings, and family backgrounds of a much larger number of women both to verify the generalizability of patterns observed in the first phase and to find patterns not represented in our smaller sample. Toward this end, two women—Sarah J. Ducey and Mary M. Malik—interviewed 87 teenage girls and their mothers, both individually and jointly, about their past and present primary attachment relationships, family situations, and other matters. In contrast to the first phase, our confidence in the reliability and validity of the information gathered from these interviews derived not from the personal relationship developed between interviewer and interviewee or from the consistency and coherence of information gathered over time, but from the fact that similar patterns emerged across women's narratives despite the identity of the interviewer and from the fact that many different trained graduate and undergraduate students reading the same interview transcript drew generally the same conclusions about what the interviewee meant to say.

My conclusions were that women in two cohorts in this population (teenage girls and their mothers) who have become pregnant as unwed teenagers differ from those who have not in at least two ways. One is with respect to their own individual and mostly unconscious ways of thinking and feeling about themselves in relationships with their parents. In the simplest terms, every daughter has a variety of conscious and unconscious goals with respect to her relationships with both parents—goals that tend to change with development. For every daughter at any given point in time, however, some goals come through louder and clearer than others. In our sample, daughters whose primary goals at the time of our interview were to get something (love, caring, closeness, special attention, material things) of which they feel they have been deprived and to ward off the anger and destructive wishes associated with feelings of deprivation were most likely to have become unwed teenage mothers. Next in line were daughters whose goals were to achieve victory over mother in a competition for father and to atone for the guilt and remorse associated with that wish. Least likely to have become unwed teenage mothers were daughters who viewed themselves as identified with mothers' values and admired ways of living and being and whose primary goals were to become autonomous and independent yet still connected adults.

The other way in which ever-pregnant teenagers differ from never-pregnant teenagers is with respect to the consistency or inconsistency of mothers' implicit and explicit communications to daughters about adolescent sexuality. Inconsistent communications from mothers are empirically associated with the adolescent pregnancy outcome for daughters, and consistent communications are associated with the never-pregnant outcome. The direction of this effect is such that communications predict pregnancy outcomes to a much greater extent than pregnancy outcomes predict communications. Inconsistent communications explicitly discourage but implicitly encourage daughters' adolescent pregnancy, whereas consistent communications both explicitly and implicitly discourage it. Mothers who say one thing and do another—for example, vehemently warn daughters of the dangers of boys lurking around every corner, but withhold information about sex, pregnancy, and birth control and/or fail to set and enforce limits on daughters' actual activities with boys—convey to daughters that they do not really mean what they say, that they really mean something else that could be the opposite of what they say.

Mothers' communications, consistent or inconsistent, reflect personal relationship goals and beliefs about what is desirable or not desirable for daughters' well-being in this sociocultural–political milieu. These beliefs derive in part from mothers' own experiences growing up in particular family environments and in part from their own experiences with adolescent sexuality. Even though all participants in this study were poor, not all family-of-origin environments were equal. They differed according to both structural and networking characteristics, some described as downwardly mobile, others as traditional, and others as upwardly mobile. Contrary to what might be expected from a strictly environmental perspective on adolescent pregnancy, variations in family environments were not directly associated with women's adolescent pregnancy outcomes in either the mother or teen cohort. Family environments, however, were indirectly associated with pregnancy outcomes through their direct associations with personal and cultural representations. A comparable indirect relationship was found between mothers' and daughters' adolescent pregnancy histories, with mothers' cultural schemas and personal representations providing the intermediate links.

Family environments and mothers' own adolescent pregnancy histories, therefore, provide contexts both for the kinds of affect-laden interactions between parents and children that are internalized in the form of mental representations of relationships and for the development of cultural schemas pertaining to adolescent sexuality and pregnancy. Whereas the ultimate motivations for adolescent pregnancy reside in the minds of mothers, daughters, and others who jointly construct personal and cultural meanings from their interactions in the immediate and larger social contexts, family environments are places in which the dynamics inherent in personal and cultural representations can be externalized, shaped and defined, and then reinternalized in new shapes and forms. Family environments are places in which psychological and sociocultural processes meet, integrate, and distill.

What This Study Does Not Mean

There are at least six things that the focus, methods, and findings of this study do not mean. First, my focus on poor African Americans in this work does not mean that adolescent pregnancy is exclusively an African American phenomenon.

Second, locating the ultimate source of people's behavior inside of their individual or collective minds is neither the same as blaming them nor the same as saying that other people or larger social contexts play no role in the construction of meanings. On the contrary, as I stated previously, meanings are always jointly constructed, beginning in the infant-mother social matrix and expanding ever-outward to include other people and social institutions. However, whereas other people and social institutions play crucial roles in the process of making meaning, meanings ultimately reside in the minds of the people who make them. Understanding what these meanings are and how they contribute to behavior is a complex and difficult process that can be short-circuited or circumvented by the act of blaming, but it is in fact the opposite of blaming (cf. Spruiell, 1989).

Third, in a related vein, what the focus on cultural and individual representations in this study does not mean is that poverty and associated conditions are unimportant variables in the adolescent pregnancy outcome. The fact that all of the participants were poor removed poverty as a variable in this study. Poverty is, of course, a constant. This fact, however, does not mean that it has no relevance or less relevance than the variables studied. On the contrary poverty insinuates itself in every facet of the adolescent pregnancy picture. It is the larger context within which other explicitly studied variables take shape and form and have their specific effects. Poverty contributes greatly to why people in this population are reluctant to abandon the formal and informal networks of support and exchange in which adolescent pregnancies and births play instrumental roles. Poverty is also a large part of the reason why many mothers recognize at some level in their minds that their own and their daughters' well-being depend to a large extent on maintaining networks and the economic, social, and emotional support the networks provide. Poverty also contributes to the facts that many families have only a single parent, that that single parent may have to work two jobs if she is lucky enough to have any job at all, and that that single parent may be severely stressed, prone to emotional problems or substance abuse, or otherwise less able to adequately parent her children. Children growing up in poor single-parent homes are more likely to develop the kinds of internal representations of parental relationships that are associated with adolescent pregnancy outcomes.

At the same time, poverty does not inevitably lead to unwed adolescents' pregnancies, as demonstrated by the girls and women in this study who have not followed that path. Further, the eradication of poverty, if this were possible, would not speedily eliminate the unwed teenage pregnancy behavior pattern. This is because unconscious representations, once developed, do not change easily, even when the contexts in which they originally developed change. Moreover, mothers' unconscious representations developed over many years continue to constitute contexts for the development of their children's unconscious representations, even when social and economic contexts change. Changing contexts to support alternative adaptations and representational developments on the parts of individuals and groups, however, can promote a gradual shift to different patterns of behavior, especially if individuals and families can be helped to become more aware of the representations that mitigate against changes in behavior. This point of view emphasizes the difficulty and complexity of the task but also its hopefulness if policymakers can become acquainted with and open to the idea that social problems with multiple causes require interventions at multiple levels of the individual–social spectrum. If, on the contrary, psychological issues are ignored in both research and formulations of policy, then expectations for change based on social or economic interventions will be unrealistically high, interventions will most likely fail, and some will be led to conclude that the problems are intractable and not worth addressing. Rather than working to the detriment of poor African American families, then, attention to psychological issues *is* necessary to avoid the kinds of distortions that critics of the psychological–developmental perspective most fear.

Fourth, what the focus on cultural and individual representations in this research does *not* mean is that these personal representations or

modes of communication are unique to poor African American populations. As much work in the psychological literature with both clinical and
nonclinical populations has shown, people have similar unconscious relationship goals, and parents sometimes communicate mixed messages to
children regardless of racial, ethnic, socioeconomic, or national identities.
What is different in different contexts is how these relationship dynamics
and modes of communication get played out. Poverty is clearly one aspect
of a context in which certain kinds of relationship dynamics get played
out in the form of adolescent pregnancies; another is historical tradition.
As I describe in chapter 2, teenage pregnancies have served networking
functions for poor African Americans since precolonial West African
times. The history of adolescent pregnancy in this population makes it a
more viable and culturally acceptable expression of relationship goals than
in some others.

Fifth, what a focus on mothers in this research does not mean is that
fathers are unimportant figures in daughters' adolescent pregnancy outcomes. Although mothers are foregrounded to a much greater extent than
fathers in this research, it is understood that mothers' and daughters'
intrapsychic and interpersonal relationships with each other always
develop and are played out in the contexts of relationships with men
(fathers, husbands, boyfriends). At all developmental levels, mothers'
thoughts and feelings about daughters and daughters' thoughts and feelings about mothers, both conscious and unconscious, are very much influenced by the availability of fathers and husbands and the specific
relationships that women have with men both intrapsychically and interpersonally. That men appear mostly in the background of things in this
book has more to do with their inaccessibility to me as a researcher than
with their relative importance in the adolescent pregnancy phenomenon.

Sixth, what my focus on poor African Americans from a White, middle-class perspective does not mean is that I believe we are not different
or that somehow I can erase the differences by putting myself in their
place. At the same time, all is not lost in the attempt of one person to
understand others, no matter how different they may be, if that one person can be clear about her own perspective, cognizant of when and how
that perspective enters into her formulation of others' meanings, and
aware at all times that alternative formulations of others' meanings are
always possible. I point out in chapter 6 of this book:

> The more one knows about something, the easier it is to find it,
> and the more meaning can be attributed to it once it is found. We
> acknowledge, however, that at the same time that prior knowl-
> edge of patterns and processes facilitates finding and under-
> standing them, it can also obscure discovery of other possible

patterns and processes. The very fact that cluster analyses of principal component scores can produce numerous sets of patterns from the same data, and people looking at these various patterns through different theoretical lenses can attribute different meanings, leaves open the possibility that the cluster solutions we have chosen and the interpretations we will make may not be the only possible ways of understanding mothers' and daughters' representations.

The same caveat applies not only to interpretations of mothers' and daughters' representations, but also to the overall pattern of findings "discovered" and interpreted in this research. In this regard, however, the adage "seek and ye shall find" applies to some extent regardless of the specific theoretical or disciplinary viewpoint of the researcher. Whether the formulations I offer in this book are right or wrong and whether they accurately approximate what is "really" going on will be judged by whether they lead now or later to the opening up of new ideas, to a new way of thinking about old ideas, or to a new or clearer way of putting old ideas together.

In sum, this research illustrates that the phenomenon of unwed adolescent pregnancy in this poor, African American population is like a tree with deep roots in the past, deep roots in the present culture, and deep roots in the unconscious recesses of people's minds. The tree also has branches that reach into the larger society and the conditions there that keep people poor, undereducated, and otherwise disadvantaged. Although the roots are mostly out of sight and the branches are in plain view, any serious attempt to understand the growth and development of the tree must take account of both.

Acknowledgments

Four people were indispensable to the success of this research. I mention them here in chronological order of their appearance in the project. The first is Martha Ward, Research Professor of Anthropology at the University of New Orleans, and author of *Them Children: A Study in Language Learning*, the book that inspired my interest and belief in the possibilities of ethnographic research. From beginning to end, Martha was unwavering in her support. She humored, encouraged, instructed, advised, corrected, consoled, commiserated and celebrated with me, and for all these things I am forever grateful.

The second person is Henry Reiff, now an associate professor of special education at Western Maryland College in Westminster, Maryland, who came with me to the field site for the first year of the ethnographic phase. Without Henry, I would not have had the courage or the perspective I needed to persist in the participant observation methodology in the face of what often seemed to be insurmountable obstacles and set-backs. With good humor, imagination, and willingness to try almost anything, Henry was the mainstay of this project in the early months.

The third and fourth persons are my collaborators and good friends, Mindy (Mary M.) Malik and Sarah Ducey. Mindy and Sarah were graduate students at the University of New Orleans who worked with me in the second phase of the project and whose doctoral dissertations are based on aspects of this research. They subsequently became cofounders of the Mercy Family Center, an agency devoted to low-cost mental health evaluation and treatment for the poor. Mindy and Sarah drove long distances every week to interview virtually all of the mothers and their teenage daughters in the larger sample; organized and supervised armies of other students and clerical help in the tasks of interview transcribing and coding and data entry and analysis; and they spent endless hours with me working to put things together in a way that made sense. The high quality of the interviews, and the extensive, detailed, and rich information we got from them, are the results of their compassion and respect for the interviewees, their interviewing acumen, and their exceptional organizational talents. Both women also made independent, creative contributions to the development and adaptation of instruments and coding schemes used in the second phase. Mindy was the prime moving force behind the conduct, theoretical conception, and coding of mother–daughter joint interviews; Sarah developed schemes for coding family environment data and participants' knowledge, attitudes, and beliefs about sex, pregnancy, and birth control.

A number of other people significantly helped me along the way. Ann McGillicuddy-Delisi, a friend and colleague in developmental psychology, performed the herculean task of reading, commenting on, and discussing in an intelligible manner an earlier, nearly unintelligible version of this manuscript. Jim Youniss, professor of developmental psychology and director of the Life-Cycle Institute at Catholic University, who has been a mentor and advocate for all of my professional life, also waded through an early version of the manuscript.

Sara Harkness and Charlie Super in their capacities as editors spent months carefully reading, re-reading, and offering constructive suggestions about the writing of the manuscript. Edward Foulks, psychoanalyst, anthropologist, and professor of psychiatry at Tulane University, read many of the adult attachment interviews and critically commented on my conceptualizations of their unconscious meanings. Vann Spruiell, my teacher, psychoanalytic supervisor, and a former editor of the *International Journal of Psycho-Analysis*, offered advice and assistance during a particularly difficult segment of this lengthy process.

Sarah Evans did an outstanding job as historian, gathering much of the material that forms the basis for chapter 2. Lynn Adams worked many hours during two summers thoughtfully reading, discussing, and coding interviews, as well as assisting in the numerous other tedious tasks involved in converting interview material to forms recognizable by computers. Phyllis Duhe, Jean Thomeczek, and Johnny Gartner meticulously transcribed interviews from audiotapes to written documents that included not only words, but the rhythms, inflections, differential emphases, and emotional concomitants of interviewees' speech. Sherry Heller helped conduct interviews and assisted with most other aspects of the second phase of research. Many other undergraduate and graduate students too numerous to name individually spent long hours reading and coding interviews and helping with clerical tasks.

Eugenia Eckert was the project director for the Office of Adolescent

Pregnancy (Department of Health and Human Welfare) grant that partially supported the second phase of this research. In addition to being a consistently enthusiastic supporter, she was at all times extremely helpful in finding extra funds for our many and varied needs.

I am grateful to Paul Stepansky of The Analytic Press for publishing this book; to John Kerr, my editor, for his astute insights, suggestions, and encouragement; and to Eleanor Kobrin and Nancy Liguori for their contributions to the production of this book.

Because of the need to protect the anonymity of the participants in this study, I cannot thank by name the principals, teachers, and other school personnel, nursing home directors, community health clinic personnel, pastors, and other members of the communities in which the study was conducted who helped in our quest to enlist and engage the cooperation of participants, and who tolerated our presence in their communities and workplaces for a long period of time. Their help was invaluable. I am especially grateful to the manager and employees of a home health agency who allowed us to use rooms in their facility rent free for many months for the purpose of conducting interviews.

Without the generosity and trust of the mothers, daughters, fathers, husbands, and boyfriends who shared their thoughts, feelings, and lives with us, this research could not have been conducted and this book could not have been written. I gratefully acknowledge their cooperation.

Finally, I would like to thank my children Eliza, Justin, and Sophie for their active support and participation in this project over the many years of its life, and for their tolerance of all the time I have spent working on my "papers." In the beginning, Justin and Sophie helped distribute flyers around the community soliciting participants. Sophie later came with me on many visits to the community and offered her very valuable 11-year-old perspective on things. Ten years later in his reincarnation as a writer, Justin read early drafts of the first few chapters and made valuable criticisms and suggestions about my writing. Eliza and Sophie, in their later reincarnations as socially conscious intelligent adults, hashed over the issues in this book with me so that I too could sound intelligent when talking about it in public. Eliza validated the whole enterprise by choosing to make qualitative research in child and family studies her life's work.

My husband Mark, who is also a psychoanalyst, spent years patiently listening to me talk about this research and read interviews out loud. His insights as to the meanings of these materials helped me over some crucial humps in the seemingly never-ending process of formulating and reformulating the ideas in this book. He was and is my harshest critic and my staunchest supporter.

1

Introduction

This book is mostly about unconscious conspiracies by poor African American girls and their mothers to promote daughters' unwed adolescent pregnancies and motherhood. It is also about mother–daughter dyads from the same population who conspire to promote a different outcome for daughters—one in which pregnancy and childbirth are delayed beyond adolescence and occur in the context of marriage. In the background of both conspiracies are men—fathers, boyfriends, and husbands—who, whether actually present in women's lives or not, set the stage for the kinds of interpersonal and intrapsychic relationships that mothers and daughters forge with one another and, as a consequence, for the ultimate outcomes of daughters' adolescent sexual activities.

The idea that adolescent pregnancy is a problem to be studied originated with the poor, African American women living in a sugarcane-growing region of southern Louisiana known as the River Parishes. I first visited this region in 1985 with Henry Reiff, then a graduate student in special education, with the goal of finding a naturalistic setting in which to study the development of moral concepts in children. To enlist families for our study, Henry and I distributed flyers to people's houses announcing that we were university teachers interested in studying how children learn right from wrong and that we would be willing to tutor children having trouble in school in exchange for being able to spend a few hours per week observing their day-to-day interactions with peers and adults. Several families responded with interest, and we made arrangements to start right away.

It quickly became apparent that the women we talked to were less interested in having their children tutored or in how children learn right from wrong than in the more immediate problem of how poor they were and how they felt unable to raise themselves up out of this dismal economic situation. We became intrigued by what seemed to be a clear contradiction between women's stated beliefs that adolescent pregnancy is detrimental to economic advancement and their behavior of continuing this pattern of childbirth. After a few months, we had turned our attention away from the study of moral concept development to the question of why girls in this community continue to become pregnant as unwed adolescents.[1]

From the conscious perspectives of women who had become mothers as adolescents, adolescent pregnancies were unwanted. They had "just happened," had happened because of ignorance about how babies are conceived, or had happened because methods for preventing or aborting pregnancies were either unknown or inaccessible. One older woman recounted how, as a 14-year-old girl, she walked past the house of an older man (in his 30s) every day on her way to school. After a while, they started "talking," and one thing led to another. When she realized she was pregnant, she told her friends, and they said "Oooh, your Mama's gonna kill you." To avert this calamity, she drank an entire bottle of castor oil, hoping this would abort the fetus. Although she knew about other methods of "throwing babies away" (a concoction she called "Blue Stone" and the services of midwives), neither of these seemed immediately accessible; she had heard of Blue Stone but did not know where to get it and did not want to ask, and the midwives lived on the other side of town. Inadvertently, the empty bottle of castor oil was left lying out where Mama could find it. Mama did find it, and in a predicted rage, banished the daughter to her older sister's house for several months. The story had a happy ending, however, with mother relenting and agreeing to raise the

---

[1] The adults and adolescents I talked to in this phase of the study—from whose stories I derived the tentative hypotheses stated at the end of chapter 3—all knew the purpose of my visits and what I intended to do with the information they gave me. When I decided to change the focus of my study from moral concept development to adolescent pregnancy, I directly and explicitly informed the people I knew best at that time. I asked their permission to include my observations and interviews with them in a book about why girls get pregnant as teenagers. I explained that anything they told me or that I observed would be written in such a way that other people could not identify them. People readily and uniformly agreed to my request; indicated that they too wanted to know why girls keep getting pregnant as teenagers; and seemed both bemused and flattered by my interest in their lives, thoughts, and opinions. As I met more people later on, I always explained myself and my presence there by stating that I was writing a book about why girls get pregnant as teenagers. My requests for informal interviews about adolescent pregnancy and related topics were further specific reminders of my purpose.

People asked me questions about what I was finding out and about how my book was coming. The first question I welcomed as an indication that people understood my purpose and as a way of testing my current speculations. The second question I answered truthfully by stating that my book was still in the mental planning stage.

baby and daughter eventually meeting and marrying a man with whom she lived for the rest of her life.

The baby, in the meantime, grew up to become an unwed adolescent mother at age 15. Her story was of meeting a man while out walking with her friends. They started "talking," and again, one thing led to another. When she first told us her story, this woman insisted that when she was a teenager, she thought babies came down the river by barge and that she had been completely taken by surprise when her own first baby arrived by a different venue. A few years later, however, when reminded of this belief, she recanted and admitted just telling us this because she thought that was what we wanted to hear. Her real reason for becoming pregnant, she said then, was because she was ready to have a baby.

We were skeptical about these conscious theories of former adolescent mothers. On the one hand, although we believed that women believed that adolescent pregnancies had "just happened" as they described, we also believed that behavior that seems to have just happened always has multiple motivational sources. Although these motives may not be consciously known by the persons involved, the goal of research is to discover and describe them.

We were just as skeptical of the idea that the younger women in this community do not know how babies are made or how the making of babies can be prevented. Although the older women we talked to were teenagers before the days of school-based health education programs or widespread availability of birth control, this was clearly not the case for the younger women, who for the most part had become adolescent mothers within the last decade. As we were to learn later in the study, the public schools and health clinics in the River Parishes have been active for at least a decade in promoting sex (health) education and the accessibility of contraceptives. Movies and pamphlets about sex, pregnancy, and contraceptives are routine components of health education programs beginning in fifth grade; health clinics are conveniently located near schools; and the schools grant permission for students to leave campus during school hours for visits to the clinic.

Further, even small children we talked to had some knowledge about sex, how babies are made, and birth control—ideas they uninhibitedly shared. One 4$^{1}/_{2}$-year-old girl I tutored in the beginning of our study, for example, invited me in our first session to inspect the little white pills her mother kept in the refrigerator that stopped her from having babies and that made her "tizzies" get big. Six- and 7-year-old boys whom we "interviewed" in the context of our moral development study told stories about "bad" men who "messed with" their sisters and who should therefore be arrested and put in jail for life. These spontaneous comments, we thought, revealed a normal childhood interest in babies and sex and an environment in which open discussion of such matters is allowed. Under these circumstances, we thought it unlikely that older girls and women were ignorant about sex and pregnancy.

Our own theories, meanwhile, were developing along different lines. One very powerful motive for unwed adolescents' pregnancies in this community, we hypothesized, might have to do with tradition. Many girls getting pregnant as adolescents in this community, it seemed, were doing what their ancestors in precolonial West Africa had done; what their slave ancestors who lived and worked the same plantations in this region had done; and more immediately, what their older sisters, mothers, grandmothers, and great-grandmothers had done. Most immediately, adolescents getting pregnant in this community were doing what many other girls in their peer group were doing. With this tradition behind and around them, what else could girls do?

A second possible motive, we thought, might have to do with how poor these families were. Although most teens and young adults had completed or were in the process of completing their high school educations or G.E.D.s (Graduation Equivalency Degrees), going to college cost money they did not have. Jobs in this region for poor African American men or women, regardless of whether they had a diploma, were few and far between. Moreover, for reasons that were unclear at the time, job prospects that did materialize always seemed to fall through. Survival in this environment of limited prospects seemed to depend on the social and economic support provided by kin and extra-kin networks. Because it seemed clear from our initial observations that babies of unwed mothers were a focal point of networking activities, we surmised that adolescent pregnancies might play a role in keeping these networks together. What that role might be remained to be seen.

A third possible reason why girls get pregnant in this community, we suspected, might have to do with their mothers. On an interpersonal front, mothers' emotional and verbal reactions to daughters' entrances into puberty were so forceful and intense that, although the mothers explicitly encouraged daughters to abstain from sexual activity, the reactions seemed to have the opposite effect. These patterns of actions and reactions by mothers and daughters, moreover, were "scripted" in that they seemed to recur in standard form among mother–daughter dyads throughout the community. We speculated that these standard scripts have developed over historical time in this population and are learned anew by successive generations of adolescent girls through interactions with mothers. On an intrapsychic front, the stories that both mothers and daughters told suggested that becoming pregnant and bearing a child as an unwed adolescent served some unconscious purposes for the mother–daughter relationship. It seemed, therefore, that mothers, having one foot in the sociocultural and the other in the psychological–developmental compartments of daughters' internal representational worlds, must play a key role in daughters' adolescent pregnancies.

At the same time, however, there were older women, younger women, and girls in this community who had not become or were not currently pregnant as adolescents. These women had the same ancestry, were just as poor, and seemed to live in the same kinds of family environments as women who had become adolescent mothers. Moreover, not all daughters talked about or interacted with their mothers in the same way. The task of understanding why some adolescent girls get pregnant and others do not; how to sort out these possible reasons; and once sorted, how to fit them back together in some coherent framework soon became our central goal.

The specific questions we had in mind at this initial juncture, then, had to do with both sociocultural and psychological–developmental motives for adolescent pregnancies among poor, unwed African Americans. What are the cultural motives? What are the psychological motives? Are both kinds of motives important, or does one category supersede the other? How can we assess cultural and psychological motives, especially if the people themselves are not consciously aware of them? If both kinds of motives are important, how can we understand the relations among them? Can an understanding of these relations in the present day help us to understand how the adolescent pregnancy system in this population has changed and is changing?

In addressing these questions throughout this research, I bring to bear a set of diverse psychological and anthropological theoretical perspectives that, in one form or another, are concerned with the interplay in complex systems of human behavior between psychological and cultural motivations. These theoretical perspectives differ, among other ways, with respect to the degree to which cultural and psychological motives are granted separate reality status and with respect to their conceptualizations of relations between culture and psychology. My primary goal in simultaneously applying these perspectives to my observations about adolescent pregnancy is not to choose among them, but to construct a view of the adolescent pregnancy system that is more comprehensive than any perspective alone can provide.

In the remainder of this chapter, I first explain why more research on the well-studied topic of adolescent pregnancy is needed and then briefly review the theories that helped me to understand adolescent pregnancy in this rural, African American population.

WHY MORE RESEARCH ON ADOLESCENT PREGNANCY IS NEEDED

The Problem

There are two primary reasons why adolescent pregnancy is increasingly viewed as a problem in our society. One is illustrated in Figure 1-1, which shows that birth rates to unmarried teenagers of all races combined have steadily increased since at least 1970 (Ventura, Martin, Mathews, & Clarke, 1996). Closer inspection of the figure shows that these increases are largely due to increases in rates for Whites.[2] Rates for African Americans remained more or less stable between 1970 and 1994, with the 1994 rate only slightly higher than the 1970 rate. Whereas in 1970, birth rates to unmarried African American teenagers were almost 10 times as high as for Whites, the difference had narrowed by 1994 to only three times the rate for Whites.[3] In other words, unmarried White teenagers have been increasingly likely since 1970 to give birth to a child, whereas the trend for African Americans has undulated within a fairly narrow range with the overall slope remaining flat. The increasing visibility of adolescent pregnancy as a social problem, then, must partly be attributed to overall trends in the White population.

The second reason why adolescent pregnancy is increasingly viewed as a problem in our society can be inferred from Figure 1-2. Since 1940, the context for teenage pregnancies in both the Black and White populations has changed dramatically. Whereas in 1940, two-thirds of Black teenagers and 93% of White teenagers becoming pregnant did so in the context of marriage, in 1994 nearly all (96%) Black teenagers and 68% of White teenagers becoming pregnant were not married (Ventura et al., 1995, 1996). This change in the mating habits of teenagers of both races has been accompanied by increases in a host of other social problems that disproportionately plague families living in poverty, and especially poor African American families who are the continuing targets of racial discrimination. These problems include joblessness, drug usage, single par-

---

[2] Ventura, Taffel, Mosher, Wislong and Henshaw (1995) suggested that increases in rates for White teenagers can be partially explained by the relatively high rates for Hispanic women and the growing proportion of births to Hispanic women. Because about one fifth of births categorized to White women are to Hispanic women, high rates for the latter affect the overall White rate. The nonmarital birth rate for non-Hispanic White women of all ages in 1994 was 20.8, as compared to 25.4 when Hispanic White women are included.

[3] In 1994, 32.6% of all live births were to unmarried women, 25.4% for Whites (including Hispanic Whites), and 70.4% for African Americans. Also in 1994, 13.1% of all births were to women younger than 20, 11.3% for Whites, and 23.2% for African Americans (Ventura et al., 1996).

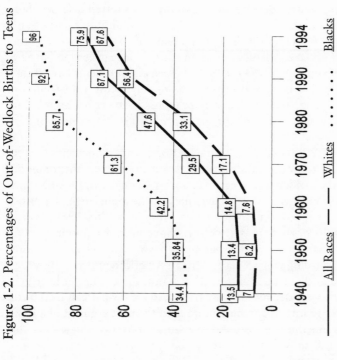

Figure 1-2. Percentages of Out-of-Wedlock Births to Teens

— All Races — — Whites · · · · · Blacks

Note. Data were taken from Ventura et al. (1995, 1996). These rates reflect the numbers of live births per 1,000 individuals in an Age x Race subgroup.

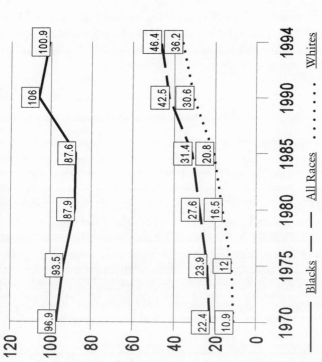

Figure 1-1. Birth Rates to Unmarried Teens

— Blacks — — All Races · · · · · Whites

Note. Data were taken from Ventura et al. (1995, 1996). These rates reflect the numbers of live births per 1,000 individuals in an Age x Race subgroup. Preliminary data for 1995 from the National Center for Health Statistics indicate that the birth rate for African American unmarried teenagers has dropped again to 95.5 births per 1,000 women from 100.9 in 1994 (Rosenberg et al., 1996). This continues a downward trend that has been in effect since 1991.

ent households, welfare dependency, sexually transmitted diseases, failure to complete a high school education, and poor health for mothers and infants. Together with the increasing availability of contraceptives and the skyrocketing costs of entitlement programs for teenage girls who have no other source of support (Ladner, 1987), these social problems have transformed what once was viewed benignly as merely a cultural variant on mating, childrearing, and childbearing practices in the Black population into what is now viewed as a major social problem in urgent need of correction (Nathanson, 1991).

In the past 20 years, much time, effort, and money have been expended trying to understand the adolescent pregnancy phenomenon and to reduce the incidence of such pregnancies among African Americans and other ethnic groups. As researchers now acknowledge (e.g., Dryfoos, 1990; Musick, 1993; Polit, 1986, 1989; Polit & White, 1988; Ward, 1991), the results of these massive efforts have been disappointing. On the one hand, scholars have yet to get much beyond surface explanations and intuition regarding why so many African American girls become pregnant as unwed adolescents. On the other hand, there is as yet little evidence that the recent declines in unmarried African American teen birth rates since 1991 represent anything more than the next segment of a basically flat trend line that has been moving within a narrow range since the 1970s or that this downward trend will be any more permanent or sustainable than the earlier decline seen in the period between 1970 and 1985. Indeed, as I discuss in the last chapter of this book, there are more reasons than not to predict increases rather than decreases in African American unmarried teen birth rates in future years.

Trends in Research and Intervention

Rather than focusing on problems of prevention, subsequent pregnancies, and the sociopsychological roots of adolescent pregnancy, intervention programs have focused primarily on adolescent girls who are already raising babies and on "feel good" support services that appeal to politicians under pressure to do something about the social ills of the inner city (Ward, 1991). Model and demonstration programs have taken as their mission the goal of linking adolescent mothers with existing educational, social, and health services, including "counseling, daycare, G.E.D. preparation, job training, parenting skills, nutrition supplements, referrals within bureaucracies and tickets to zoos, movies, or other public entertainments" (Ward, 1991, p. 7). Although these programs have improved the quality of life for adolescent girls and their babies, they have not substantially decreased unwed pregnancy rates.

In similar fashion, research has tended to focus more on the consequences of adolescent pregnancy for girls and their children than on precursors (cf. recent reviews by Brooks-Gunn & Chase-Landale, 1991; Brooks-Gunn & Furstenberg, 1986; Osofsky, Hann, & Peebles, 1993). The presumption that adolescent mothers beget adolescent mothers has led to the assumption that consequences of adolescent pregnancy in one generation of women are antecedents for the next. Both the presumption and the assumption, however, have been challenged by findings that adolescent mothers do not necessarily beget adolescent mothers (Furstenberg, Brooks-Gunn & Morgan, 1987; Furstenberg, Levine & Brooks-Gunn, 1990) and that adolescent pregnancies per se do not necessarily put lower income African American girls or their offspring at risk for long-term socioeconomic disadvantage (Geronimus & Korenman, 1991).

A second trend has been the reluctance to acknowledge the multifaceted and complex nature of the adolescent pregnancy phenomenon. Researchers and program planners alike have tended to focus on isolated correlates of adolescent pregnancy, such as poverty, low self-esteem, depression, undereducation, ignorance or inaccessibility of contraceptives, lack of parental guidance, or lack of role models without delving into the more perplexing problems of how and where these variables fit into an overall contextual framework or exactly how these individual characteristics might lead or motivate an adolescent girl to become an unwed mother. On the contrary, correlations are most often presented as de facto evidence of the motivational force of the so-called independent variable. Rarely are researchers moved to ask why other girls in other contexts possessing the same characteristics (e.g., poverty, depression, low self-esteem, and the like) do not become pregnant as adolescents. Although these individual variables may well constitute important pieces of the adolescent pregnancy puzzle for all ethnic groups, the puzzle itself still remains in pieces.

A third related trend has been a selective focus on sociocultural correlates of adolescent pregnancy to the neglect of deep-level psychological–developmental factors (Musick, 1993). Psychological studies that have had some impact on program planning are those that focus on experience-near constructs such as self-esteem (Held, 1981; Koniak-Griffen, 1989; B. C. Miller, Cristensen, & Olson, 1978; Pattern, 1981; Vernon, Green, & Frothingham, 1983; Zongker, 1977) or self-efficacy (Dunst, Vance, & Cooper, 1986; Meyerowitz & Malev, 1973; Ralph, Lochman, & Thomas, 1984; Segal & DuCette, 1973; Walters, Walters, & McKenry, 1986). The empirical connections between both of these measures and adolescent pregnancy have proved to be tenuous, yet both continue to receive much attention by program developers and the media (Ward, 1991). On the other hand, clinically based studies (e.g., Barglow, 1968; Bibring, Dwyer, Huntington, & Valenstein, 1961; Blos, 1962, 1967; Deutsch, 1944, 1967; Ornstein & Ornstein, 1985; Osofsky, Osofsky, & Diamond, 1988) that address the unconscious dynamic reasons why adolescent girls wish to become pregnant—what Musick (1993) termed the "inner realities that govern (the adolescent girl's) response" (p. 9) to demands and opportunities in her environment—have been ignored by researchers and policymakers alike.

Explanations most often given for discounting studies of unconscious motivation are that the studies are necessarily based on small samples, utilize "unscientific" clinical techniques for gathering data, and interpret findings in the context of psychoanalytic theory—a framework that at best has met with mixed reviews in the fields of sociology, anthropology, and psychology. Other reasons for the neglect of deeper level psychological motives for adolescent pregnancy were suggested by Musick (1993):

> The broader debate about how best to address persistent poverty in families and to renew healthy social life in the communities where these families live has tended to gloss over the developmental and psychological factors associated with phenomena such as adolescent childbearing. Although the notion that psychological difficulties can lead to lower social and work-related functioning and downward mobility among middle-class people is generally accepted, there is resistance to this notion in regard to poor people. Perhaps such a notion carries an unwelcome message about the complexity and deep-rooted nature of these problems; perhaps it outwardly resembles the now discredited "culture of poverty" perspective. For many people, attention to psychological issues implies a blame-the-victim viewpoint, calling for psychotherapeutic approaches to people simply because they are poor. Or perhaps the reluctance to look at personal issues stems from a common reluctance to look inward for fear of stirring up repressed feelings and vulnerabilities. Developmental and psychological issues are, after all, universal human phenomena. Touching these issues in others, we risk touching them in ourselves. Better to substitute a litany of social and economic horrors; better to keep telling the same sensational stories of crime and drugs and family violence and teen pregnancy and educational and economic disaster. (p. 13)

One reason why it is important to ask questions about the psychological–developmental and cultural motives for adolescent pregnancy and their interrelations, therefore, is because these questions are critical for understanding and for program-planning. As yet, these questions have not been adequately addressed in the adolescent pregnancy literature. Exploration at "deeper, more analytic levels of inquiry" (Musick, 1993, p. 14) about both cultural and psychological motives is needed to understand the adolescent pregnancy system. At the same time, these deeper level inquiries must be combined with larger-sample methodologies designed to empirically study the complex relations among cultural and psychological variables. In the research reported in this book, deep-level analytic inquiries were conducted into both cultural and psychological –developmental motives for adolescent pregnancy in the ethnographic phase, and then followed with an extension of the research into a larger sample of women from the same population. Both of these phases of the research were indispensable in understanding why lower income African American girls in this population become pregnant as unwed adolescents.

RELATION TO THE GENERAL QUESTION OF WHY PEOPLE DO WHAT THEY DO

In asking these specific questions about the cultural and psychological motives underlying adolescent pregnancy and their interrelationships, this book also addresses a more general issue of concern to both psychologists and anthropologists. What motivates people in a given population or culture to put so much effort into doing some things rather than doing other things (D'Andrade, 1992)? Why, for example, do so many lower income African American girls become pregnant as unwed adolescents rather than delaying pregnancy until they are older and married? In asking this more general question, therefore, I enter a debate, which has preoccupied cultural anthropologists and psychologists for a long time, over whether it is necessary to invoke both individual psychological and cultural constructs in explaining socially significant action patterns, and if so, how to understand the systemic relations between these two categories of constructs.

The theoretical perspectives pertinent to this debate, including those brought to bear on our understanding of the adolescent pregnancy system in this research, can be arranged along a continuum defined by the degree to which cultural and psychological sources of motivation are granted separate reality status. At one end of the continuum are heterogeneous groups of theories that blur the distinction between cultural and psychological sources or assume that one is superfluous or superseded by the other (e.g., the cultural relativism of Mead and Benedict, in which individual psychological variables were subsumed by cultural, and the psychobiological reductionism of Roheim, in which culture was seen as a reflection of unconscious, dynamic conflicts). A modern-day representative of this end of the continuum is Shweder (e.g., Shweder & Sullivan, 1990), who, in Strauss's (1992) words, contended that "behavior follows the curves of culturally defined realities and no other forces (of material interests or repressed needs, for example) are required to explain why we do what we do" (p. 13). Most people in American middle-class culture, Shweder argued, would react negatively to a weed and take action to remove it from their flower gardens. The motive to eradicate weeds is built into the culturally constituted "weed schema," and from this perspective, there is no need to invoke individual psychological motives.

On the opposite end of the continuum are those positions that treat cultural and psychological sources of motivation as distinct but interacting processes in sociopsychological systems. Such a position is taken, for example, by LeVine (1982) in his evolutionary theory of culture and personality. Socially significant action patterns in a population, said LeVine, simultaneously are responsive to sociocultural norms and unconscious psychological needs and wishes of individuals. Unconscious needs and wishes, said LeVine, develop in early childhood and are primarily accidental by-products of social stimuli impinging on children. These social stimuli are by-products of sociostructural features of family environments, the latter of which are adaptations to ecological niches in which people live. Sociocultural norms are culturally constructed, agreed-upon ways of living, thinking, and feeling that originate because of their primary adaptive value but that in time may take on additional, secondary functions. Socially significant action patterns, LeVine suggested, are compromise solutions to the often competing demands and opportunities of these cultural and psychological sources, or to what Spiro (1961) termed duty and desire.

Dialectical Viewpoints

Somewhere between these two extreme positions is a third that takes a dialectical perspective on the relation between individual psychological and sociocultural sources of motivation for socially significant action patterns. At various points in our research, we made use of three theoretical positions that implicitly adhere to a dialectical perspective in thinking about complex systems of human behavior. These were the psychoanalytic theory of Hans Loewald (1980), the cognitive anthropological theory of D'Andrade (1990, 1992, 1993; Strauss, 1992), and the attachment theory of Bowlby (1973; Bretherton, 1985; Main, Kaplan, & Cassidy, 1985). Although there are real, irreducible differences among these points of view, all have in common a mutual rejection of fundamental Cartesian dualisms in favor of a view of individual and social as interdependent poles of single wholes—irreducible facts of dialectical reality—that contain within themselves the essential conditions for change.

Attachment theory. Attachment theorists, for example, have in recent years paid considerable attention to cultural as well as individual psychological meanings of patterns of attachment behavior (e.g., Bretherton, 1985; Harwood, 1992; Harwood, Miller, & Lucca-Irizarry, 1995). Although an explicit theory of individual/social relations has not emerged within this paradigm, both personal and cultural meanings are assumed to be components of the same mental representations of attachment relationships, or what attachment theorists term *internal working models* (Bowlby, 1973). Caregivers serve the dual functions of creating contexts for particular qualities of interpersonal experience for children and of conveying cultural meanings regarding these experiences. Both kinds of meanings—individual and cultural—are internalized simultaneously in children's working models of self in relationship to others. Internalization, in attachment theory (e.g., Bretherton, 1985, 1990, 1991) is a process of constructing, differentiating, and integrating representations of interactive events with caregivers, including associated feelings and sensations.

Loewald's psychoanalytic theory. Like attachment theory, Loewald's theory proposes that individual psychological and cultural meanings are created jointly through interactions in the infant–mother, later child–adult, matrices and focuses explicitly on the internalizing–externalizing processes whereby internality and externality are gradually created in these matrices. As Loewald (1980) put it:

> It is one of its characteristics that psychoanalytic psychology does not view the psychic life of the individual in isolation, but in its manifold relations and intertwinings with other spheres and aspects of life, such as social–cultural life and the somatic–biological sphere. It tends to see these as reflected in and as reflections of the individual psyche; and in these respects, they are within the realm of psychoanalytic investigation. (p. 70)

Like attachment theorists, Loewald acceded an essential role in the process of psychic structure formation to parents. He stated that

> what from an external (i.e., nonpsychoanalytic) observer's point of view are called objects (parents), are indispensable and crucial factors in the organization of psychic functioning and psychic structure . . . and what is naively called subject (infant, child) plays an essential part in the organization of objects (not merely of object representations). (p. 127)

Thus, Loewald suggested that an important part played by parents is to help organize and define infants' earliest experiences, both inner (e.g., bodily urges, kinesthetic sensations, feelings, etc.) and outer (sources of stimulation coming from the external world of people and objects). These experiences jointly created in the infant–mother and later child–adult–societal matrices are internalized over the course of development as the child's own. In this study, Loewald's views about the internalization process were particularly apropos to my understanding of mothers' and daughters' representations of their relationships—a key component of the adolescent pregnancy model that ultimately emerged from the research.

Cognitive anthropological viewpoints. Cognitive anthropologists and psychologists, in contrast to attachment and psychoanalytic theorists, emphasize culturally constituted cognitive schemas (schemas arrived at jointly over historical time by members of a culture and shared by at least some individuals in that culture) and assert their primacy in motivational systems over universal needs and drives such as hunger, sex, and aggression. The theoretical argument presented by D'Andrade (1993) is as follows:

> (1) (Culturally constituted) schemas, which form the reality-defining system of the human, provide information about what states of the world can and should be pursued;
> (2) Because of the centrality of schemas in determining appropriate action, top-level schemas (e.g. love and work) tend to function as goals;
> (3) Drives, affects, and other kinds of instigations to action function by activating goal-schemas, not by instigating behavior directly, since for humans appropriate action depends on role and setting contexts which require elaborate cognitive interpretation prior to action. (p. 33)

Questions asked by cognitive anthropologists are also about internalization. How do people make the public information that they are exposed to into their own thought-feelings? What is the nature of this process through which frequently conflicting, inconsistent, and sometimes only implicit social messages become experienced by individuals as relatively coherent thoughts and feelings of their own? How is it that some cultural constructs acquire motivational force for some individuals in a culture but not for others? Cognitive anthropologists, like attachment theorists, give answers to these questions that reflect a preference for thinking about individuals' thought-feelings as having origins in external events or interactions. D'Andrade (1993) implied, for example, that the individual's internal world is largely constituted by hierarchies of socially and culturally constituted schemas, learned primarily through shaping in early socialization experiences. And citing Sperber (1985), Strauss (1992) said that "social action is the result of a process by which public events are turned into private representations and then acted on, thereby creating new public events" (p. 16). For these theorists, then, the individual psyche is reflected in and a reflection of culturally and socially constituted models of reality.

USE OF THEORY AND PLAN OF THE BOOK

The specific problems and hypotheses that became the focus of our research were not invented ahead of time, but were discovered in the early months of the study. I began this study, however, with theoretical biases reflecting my training in developmental psychology and psychoanalysis. These biases are manifested in five domains. First, I chose to focus on the goal of understanding adolescent pregnancy not as an isolated phenomenon, but as one process in a coherent, unified system. Second, I believe that although adolescent pregnancy is not exclusively an African American phenomenon, it is a different phenomenon in the African American population than the White population—one with different historical and social origins and thereby different meanings for individuals involved (cf. McAdoo, 1988b; Ogbu, 1981; Washington, 1982). The third bias is manifested in my search for multiple meanings of the adolescent pregnancy behavior pattern—meanings that are conscious and unconscious; meanings residing within the individual, the family group, and the culture; and meanings that satisfy individual wishes and desires as well as moral goals. Fourth, I recognized early on in the study that the appropriate unit of analysis in a study of adolescent pregnancy is not the adolescent girl per se, but the girl in relationship with significant attachment figures. The fifth bias underscores my belief that accounting for adolescent pregnancy in its present forms, as LeVine (1982) suggested, means reconstructing its history within the individual and within the culture, as well as elucidating its contemporary social and psychological meanings.

Formal theory entered into my conceptualization of the adolescent pregnancy system only after I was well into the process of gathering ethnographic material. This material, as discussed in chapter 3, was filled with seeming contradictions and paradoxes. Two of LeVine's (1982) propositions were of particular help in making sense out of these contradictions: One is that phenotypic (frequently recurring) behavior patterns in a population are jointly determined by often competing individual psychological and sociocultural–historical forces, the latter which are mutually constructive of each other; the other is that motives for behavior in both individual psychological and sociocultural realms are both conscious and unconscious, explicit and implicit. These propositions helped me to understand the dynamics underlying the evolution of mating and childbearing practices in the African American population reviewed in chapter 2, and they played a significant background role in my formulation of an informal theory of adolescent pregnancy described in chapter 3. On the basis of this theoretical framework, I formulated specific hypotheses and questions about adolescent pregnancy that were addressed in the larger-sample interview phase to follow.

In chapters 4 through 8, I describe the larger-sample interview phase and the ways in which a combination of quantitative and qualitative methods allowed us to first rediscover the themes in the adolescent pregnancy system I identified in the ethnographic phase and then to put them back together in a picture that in some ways looked the same but in other ways looked different. In this phase, two semistructured interviews were used to gather data about mothers' and daughters' perspectives about themselves, their relationships, and their sociocultural environments. These were the Adult Attachment Interview (AAI; George, Kaplan, & Main, 1985; Main et al., 1985) and a joint mother–daughter interview coded using a scheme developed by M. Nathanson, Baird, and Jemail (1986). On the basis of patterns discernable in individuals' responses in these interview settings, I was able to confirm and to elaborate on my conjectures with regard to the hidden (unconscious, implicit) meanings of adolescent pregnancy to women in this population.

As my conceptualization of the adolescent pregnancy system took further shape in the larger-sample interview phase, it became apparent that the influences of sociostructural and normative aspects of environments on the adolescent pregnancy pattern are mediated by the personal and cultural mental representations of individuals. These findings suggested the need for theories that directly address processes of internalization whereby interactions in the external world are reconstructed on an internal plane. Although approached from opposite ends of the spectrum, such views, as just described, are expressed in psychoanalytic, attachment and cognitive anthropological or psychological theories. Internalization processes constitute a vehicle whereby the social stimuli impinging on the child described by LeVine (1982) as well as social norms about the right and proper way to behave, become relocated from realms outside of the child to realms inside the child and the adult. As I discuss in more detail in the final chapter of this book, ignoring the internalization process accentuates the duality and separability of individuals and cultures, thus obscuring the significance of mental representation as a central integrating factor in the adolescent pregnancy system.

2

Historical Background

From the perspectives of some researchers, adolescent pregnancy in the lower income African American population is a problem in need of correction, not only for adolescent girls and their families but also for society as a whole. These researchers argue that after generations of poverty and discrimination, the African American family has become increasingly disorganized and unable to provide the traditional forms of economic and other kinds of support on which its members have so long depended (Moynihan, 1965; Rainwater & Yancey, 1967; Wilson, 1987). The rising number of pregnancies among unwed, adolescent African Americans is viewed as but one among many consequences of that trend.

A variety of explanations have been offered for the fact that adolescent girls from poor, disorganized, single-parent, undereducated, and perhaps drug-ridden homes are more likely to become unwed mothers than those from more favorable environments. Such an environment severely limits adolescents' and older individuals' prospects of forming and maintaining stable married households by limiting educational and occupational attainments (Ladner, 1988; Phipps-Yonas, 1980); reducing the number of males available for mating or who are in a position to contribute to the economic well-being of a potential family (MacLeod, 1987; Staples & Johnson, 1993); reducing the number of role models for alternative life courses (Wilson, 1987); placing obstacles in the way of parents' abilities to discipline, give advice, and otherwise assist their children in resisting the strong peer pressures toward premarital sexual activity (Brooks-Gunn & Furstenberg, 1986; Furstenberg et al., 1990; Williams, 1991); and promoting reliance on a welfare system that discriminates against stable, two-parent families. These same environments also mitigate against stable, married relationships by restricting the number of avenues that could provide adolescent girls and boys with feelings of self-worth (B. C. Miller et al., 1978; Pattern, 1981; Zongker, 1977) or self-efficacy (Meyerowitz & Malev, 1973; Ralph et al., 1984; Segal & DuCette, 1973) and by depriving adolescents of healthy emotional relationships with parents or other significant attachment figures who are themselves stressed by life circumstances (Barglow, 1968; Bierman & Bierman, 1985; Buchholz & Gol, 1986; Cobliner, 1981; Hart & Hilton, 1988; Landy, Schubert, Cleland, Clark & Montgomery, 1983; N. Miller, 1986; Schamess, 1990).

From the perspectives of other researchers, adolescent pregnancy in this same population is an adaptive strategy devised to meet girls' social, economic, and developmental needs in an environment where men, material resources, and financial resources are scarce. Having babies out of wedlock, it is argued, can help to solidify kin networks that are critical for economic and caregiving functions (Dougherty, 1978; Stack, 1974; Young, 1970), can help girls become independent and responsible and identify with their roles as women (Dougherty, 1978; Hamburg, 1986; Ladner, 1971), can allow young women time to raise children before entering the work force (Hamburg, 1986; Hogan, 1978; Ladner, 1971), can fulfill grandmothers' needs to parent (Burton, 1990), and can provide children of such mothers with a wide network of surrogate parents (Burton, 1990; Stack, 1974; Young, 1970).

Although these two perspectives seem contradictory at first, both make sense from the vantage point of history. Adolescent pregnancy may have one set of meanings for individuals in a viable, extended-family support system—historically, the traditional form of the African American family. It may have different meanings for individuals whose extended-family support system has begun to deteriorate—a relatively recent development in the history of the African American family. From this perspective, adolescent pregnancy is not a uniform phenomenon in the lower income African American population; it takes on different forms and has different meanings depending on its complex interrelations with historical, sociocultural, and individual psychological processes. Understanding adolescent pregnancy from this perspective does not mean identifying single or even multiple precursors or consequences of adolescent pregnancy; it is describing the dynamic interrelations among the components making up the larger adolescent pregnancy system.

In what follows, I present an account of the history and current state of mating and childbearing practices in this population of lower income, rural African Americans that clarifies how both of these perspectives can be true. This account suggests that adolescent pregnancy, in one form or another, has always contributed to the formation and maintenance of social networks on which members depend for their essential needs. The specific ways in which adolescent pregnancy has accomplished this networking function, as well as the forms assumed by the adolescent pregnancy behavior pattern, however, have changed over time to accommodate changes in both the proximal and distal sociocultural–political contexts of African American family life. Some of these changes in specific function and form have contributed to the increasingly problematic nature of adolescent pregnancy in some sociocultural contexts. I conclude as a result of our historical review, however, that although adolescent pregnancy may seem to be maladaptive in some contexts and adaptive in others, in fact it is both things in all contexts.

Historical Review

The psychological meanings attributed to mating and childbearing customs by individuals in past generations are not known. Thus, historical accounts of the evolution of such customs are necessarily restricted to descriptions of the customs themselves and the contexts (physical, social, political, and cultural) in which they have developed. It is tempting, given these limitations, to explain the evolution of customs solely on the basis of these sociocultural and physical contextual variables without invoking psychological meanings. One with a structuralist–functionalist viewpoint, for example, would argue that mating and childbearing customs have evolved in a particular way because external factors have channeled the choice of customs in certain directions most consistent with survival and prosperity (e.g., Fox, 1967). The custom of having babies early and frequently in nonindustrial, agrarian societies might be explained by the need to cultivate and maintain large extended families that were crucial to the survival and prosperity of individuals living in those environments.

Although it cannot be denied that mating and childbearing customs provide advantages (and disadvantages) for individuals living in certain physical or cultural environments, the observation that customs and contexts covary necessarily implies neither a functionalist view of cultural evolution nor that individual psychological meanings are not a critical component of the explanation for the evolution of customs. A dialectical systems perspective, for example, would link customs and contexts together as equally contributing components of a whole, dynamic system in which all processes are ultimately interrelated in a more or less direct fashion. Covariation from this point of view would not necessarily imply that one process is adapted to another, but that change in one brings about change in others by virtue of the disequilibrium that the first change introduces into the system as a whole. Moreover, the observation that customs work to the advantage of individuals in certain sociocultural environments does not necessarily imply that customs developed because of these advantages. Customs originally designed for one set of purposes may later come to serve other secondary purposes that work to the advantage of individuals in a particular sociocultural environment (LeVine, 1982).

Thus, although I describe here the possible advantages that mating and childbearing customs and other sociocultural institutions might have had for poor African Americans at various points in history, I do not interpret these possible advantages as explanations for these customs, but rather reserve judgment regarding explanations until these relationships as well as others can be explored more fully in subsequent chapters.

The Region

The region where this study was conducted is a stretch of land bordering both sides of the Mississippi River in the Deep South. The economy of this area has always depended heavily on the growing of sugarcane on what Whites still refer to as plantations but African Americans refer to as farms. The antebellum houses that line the river now stand in the shadow of mammoth chemical plants and oil refineries—industries that somewhat compensate when times are good for the steady decline in farming jobs for African American laborers. But when times are bad, as they have been for the petrochemical industry in the area for many years, African Americans are the first to be laid off. In the River Parishes, a high percentage of residents are poor, African American, and unemployed, and the region is distinguished by one of the highest teenage pregnancy rates in the nation.[1]

Many of the African Americans who participated in this study could trace their ancestry directly back to slaves who lived and worked on plantations in the River Parish region. Some of the members of the older generation could recall the names of their ancestors who were alive during the "Reb" days. From what little has been written about slavery in this part of the country, it can be gathered that most slaves who worked sugar plantations after the Louisiana Purchase in 1803 were imported by Americans into the region, where some of them intermarried with Creole slaves (i.e., Africans imported to Louisiana by the French or Spanish) and native Indians (Hall, 1992). The American slaves brought with them a

---

[1] In 1994, only one other state, Mississippi, and the District of Columbia had higher percentages of births to unmarried women of all races than Louisiana (42.6%). Louisiana ranked 17th in percentages of births to unmarried African American women (72.4%; Ventura et al., 1996).

slave culture that had developed over the last 2 centuries in the English colonies in the upper South and that has been described in some detail by Herskovits (1958), Gutman (1976), Frazier (1971), and others. Although there is debate over the extent to which these slaves retained aspects of their African heritage, it seems clear that continuities existed between precolonial African and slave periods in African Americans' primary allegiances to the extended family and in their patterns of mating and childbearing.

Precolonial African Societies

The many tribes from which American slaves were abducted were each collections of clans that themselves were collections of lineages, or groups of people united on the basis of a common ancestor (Fox, 1967). The members of a lineage lived together in a compound that was in close proximity to others belonging to the same clan or tribe. The vast majority of lineages in precolonial West Africa operated according to the principle of patrilineal descent, according to which a child reckoned his kinship connections through his or her father's side of the family. When a man wanted a wife in a patrilineal society, he got her from among the available women in a nearby lineage or compound; she was required to leave her own compound to reside in her husband's. Once there, she was known as "wife of the house," as opposed to "so-and-so's wife," to emphasize the importance of loyalty to the extended family as opposed to any particular man. But at the same time, she was her husband's wife and no other's. Although a man might have more than one wife, a wife had no more than one husband; she belonged to him by virtue of the fact that he had paid brideprice for her, regardless of whether they resided together in the same hut. The preferred living arrangement in most societies, in fact, was a setup in which a man had several wives who lived together with their children in separate huts and took turns visiting their common husband in his hut (Billingsley, 1968; Foner, 1975; Fox, 1967; Herskovits, 1958; Meier & Rudwick, 1976; Sowell, 1981; Sudarkasa, 1988).

In the context of these mostly patrilineal–patrilocal West African societies, patterns of reproductive behavior served necessary and important functions for the survival and prosperity of the lineage. Although customs varied among societies, it was generally the case that a man would be ready to get a wife in his mid-teens—and conversely, a woman would be ready to get a husband at the same age—and that premarital sex was a prelude to a marriage. Premarital sex in some societies was part of pubertal initiation rites or just expected as a part of the courting process. By the time a woman gave birth to a child she had conceived in this way, however, she was almost always married. Indeed, a woman's pregnancy was a happy event for a man whose primary objective was to have a wife who could bear him many children, especially sons (although daughters were good too because of the brideprice they would bring). A woman who did not become pregnant might be barren—a condition that could justify her return to her natal compound and a return of a man's brideprice. Such a fate was disastrous for a woman because the sister–daughter role was essentially useless in the patrilineal–patrilocal society. The woman's role in the society was that of wife and mother, and her value was gauged by the number of children she produced for her husband. Demonstrating her fertility at an early age was an important step by which she could enhance the prestige of herself and her husband and contribute to the continuation and perpetuation of the lineage. The extended family in West African societies performed vital economic, social, political, and military functions. Its perpetuation was critical, and procreation was considered a religious duty (Billingsley, 1968; Ladner, 1971; Meier & Rudwick, 1976; Sudarkasa, 1988).

Slavery

In the New World, lineages were disrupted, and slaves from many diverse tribes were thrown together on the same slave ship and on the same plantation. Despite the dehumanizing and disruptive conditions under which they arrived in the New World, slaves risked severe beatings, dismemberment, and death to seek relatives or marriage partners from whom they had been separated. Initially, the prospects of slaves creating new extended-family networks were poor, given the disproportionate number of male slaves and the reluctance of many slave women to bear children into slavery. Some did, however, and succeeding generations organized themselves into extended family networks that were their first line of defense against the severely depriving and dehumanizing conditions of slavery. There is a wealth of data in slave diaries and testimonies documenting various ways that consanguineal kin assisted each other with childrearing, in life crises, and in efforts to gain freedom. The same philosophy that guided African family life—"I am because We are and because We are, therefore I am" (Mbiti, 1969)—also guided the family through the horrors of slavery (Blassingame, 1972; Gutman, 1976; Ladner, 1971; Nobles, 1974; Sowell, 1981).

As in African patrilineages, the husband and wife bond in the slave family was maintained as important. Although marriage was illegal, monogamous "common-law" marriages were the norm, and the typical slave family consisted of a husband, wife, children, grandchildren, and assorted kin. As in African society, these common-law marriages were commonly but not always preceded by a premarital pregnancy and birth—the latter, as in Africa, being a prelude to a settled union. Female-headed households were a rarity and occurred only when the husband was sold or died or when the woman had children out of wedlock, often for her master, and was given her own cabin (Blassingame, 1972). The importance to women of bearing children frequently and early continued. By becoming a mother, a young woman gained the respect of her own community, a value carried to the New World by the Africans. This contributed to the perpetuation of her extended family and gave the slave master incentive not to sell her away from her extended family of origin because slave children were a highly valued economical commodity for slave owners. Thus, although the pattern of mating, childbearing, and childrearing continued in these respects, it also took on new functions that were specific to the slave situation (Bernard, 1966; Gutman, 1976; Harrison, 1988; Sudarkasa, 1988).

Emancipation to 1930

Immediately after emancipation, as many as 50% of African American Freedmen in the River Parishes left the plantations for Union army camps or for nearby cities (Grace, 1946). Some went in search of family members from whom they had been separated during slavery, others in search of urban employment which they preferred to the contracts offered them by planters under the authorization of the army of occupation and the Freedmen's Bureau. These contracts not only regulated hours and wages, but also levied fines for disobedience and stipulated that Freedmen could not leave the plantation without the permission of the employer (Cohen, 1984). African Americans were often taken advantage of because Whites wrote the contracts; most African Americans were illiterate; and, even when they could read the contracts, their lack of experience or leverage in the negotiation process rendered them powerless in changing them (Jones, 1985). Planters, in turn, considered African Americans to be undependable and an inefficient source of cheap labor. As one planter wrote to a business associate,

> [Negroes are] so saucy and unreliable that they are intolerable. [They want] their horse, their cow, their pig, and such extras a people whose time is fully paid for should not expect. Tis well some resort is left to show them the planter is not wholly dependent on their caprice, and obliged to suffer their impertinences. (Cohen, 1984, p. 119)

Yet, despite the apparent distrust and animosity felt by planters and Freedmen toward each other, many African Americans who initially fled returned to the plantations because they were generally ill-equipped to survive in urban settings.

In much of the rural Deep South, the era between the Emancipation Act of 1863 and the 1930s brought little change for African Americans in terms of real social, economic, and political opportunities, except the freedom to quit, to seek employment on another plantation, to move into the city, or to leave the state. In the political realm, African Americans had little chance to challenge the White power structure once federal forces moved out of the South. In effect, the Supreme Court's Dred Scott decision of 1857, which stated that African Americans "had no rights which the White man was bound to respect" (cited in Sowell, 1981, p. 197) remained true throughout the period (Bernard, 1966; Gutman, 1976; Jones, 1985). As in the days of slavery, Whites kept African Americans subservient and powerless during this era by effectively denying them the opportunity to become educated. When the Freedman's Bureau and the Reconstruction government withdrew from the South, public sentiment against the education of African Americans brought a swift halt to the reforms initiated after the war. By the 1920s, there were a handful of public schools for African Americans in the region, but attendance was not compulsory and only African Americans who lived within walking distance could attend. African American children who lived on plantations either were taught to read and write by literate African American tutors or received no schooling, with the result that illiteracy rates among African Americans remained exceedingly high through the 1930s (Grace, 1946).

The daily lives of African American men, women, and children during the era between the Civil War and World War II centered around their work in the sugarcane fields and their extended families. In contrast to what was happening in the Cotton Belt, where sharecropping and tenant farming among African Americans and poor Whites became increasingly prevalent between 1880 and 1930, African American men, women, and children over the age of 10 or 11 on sugar plantations continued to work the fields for wages in gangs directed by White bosses and overseers (Jones, 1985). Women and children worked in teams behind the mule-drawn wagons and ploughs driven by the African American men and were paid by the row of cane they cut and gathered. If it rained or if they were sick, they did not get paid. They earned subsistence wages or less but were able to supplement their meager resources by gardening; raising chickens and livestock; catching oppossum, rabbits, and other wildlife; fishing; and gathering and selling moss for stuffing.

As had the slaves before them, free African American laborers on the plantations lived in "quarters," rows of perhaps 10 to 20 two- or three-room cabins located along the sides of a plantation road, that functioned as self-contained communities with their own stores, churches, and cemeteries. A small number of extended families lived and worked on the same or neighboring plantations, drawing from each others' ranks for wives and husbands, but always maintaining the first-cousin incest taboo. Individual households typically consisted of mother; father; perhaps a grandparent; many children and grandchildren; and occasionally spouses of children and assorted nieces, orphans, and unrelated godchildren.

In this context, African American girls grew up knowing what was expected and that their options were limited. They knew that when they stopped being children they were expected to become adults in every sense of the word (i.e., to work, bear children, and perpetuate family ties). They knew they would become pregnant and get married and have their own cabin nearby. The order of these events did not matter much. Frequently, but not always, girls first got pregnant by an older man, a liaison that was followed shortly by marriage to a younger man that lasted a lifetime. The age of the woman at the time of her marriage varied as well, ranging from late teens and early 20s to older. Again, it did not matter much because the outcome was the same. Very young teen pregnancies were the exception and discouraged because they added an extra burden on the older women in the family and interfered with the wage-earning capacities of younger girls who could work in the fields.

When some African Americans in the older generation who can remember back to these times compare them with the present, they are inclined to say that times were better back then. To quote Emmelina, an 80-year-old former domestic servant, "Seems like there was more loving in those days, seems like there was more togetherness. . . . All the Black children and the White children would play together in the road. . . . There is togetherness now, but it's a different kind of togetherness." Another survivor of that time said, "In the quarters there was a real sense of community . . . you had your vegetable garden, your chickens, your hogs, your cow, your kin, your job. No matter how hard things were you had your place in the world."

1930 to the Present

Southern agriculture, including sugar farming in the River Parish region, was permanently altered by the Great Depression. The federal government encouraged planters to limit crop production so as to raise the price of food again. In return, the government promised funding for new machinery. Mechanization of farming decreased the need for field hands.

White landowners consolidated their holdings, displaced sharecropping families, laid off wage-earning laborers, and from then on were able to farm huge tracts of land with only a small percentage of the laborers required prior to that time. Many African American wage-earning laborers who were laid off from plantations lost not only their jobs but also their living quarters, because the latter were contingent upon employment on the plantations (Ploski & Williams, 1989).

The loss of farming jobs on sugar plantations and elsewhere coincided with two other significant events that affected African Americans throughout the South. One was World War II, which further fueled African American migration, fostered industry, and created jobs for African Americans. The second event was the Civil Rights movement that came to the River Parishes in 1962 when James Farmer rode into a town with members of CORE (Committee on Racial Equality). African Americans who were holding a meeting in a local church were teargassed by federal marshals who rode through the church on horses, ostensibly to break up the meeting. African Americans remember this with distress. According to both African Americans and Whites, poor African Americans suffered the most from this demonstration because different groups exploited them and they got nothing from it.

Changes in opportunities resulting from mechanization, World War II, and the Civil Rights movement worked both to the advantage and disadvantage of African Americans in the region. On the up side, more schools were desegregated and public transportation allowed access for all. The decrease in need for field hands freed children from work in the fields and gave them time for school. African Americans gained access to public facilities, although some places such as movie theaters and swimming pools around the region closed when African Americans gained legal access to them.

On the down side, the loss of farming jobs and migrations of people out of the region resulted in deterioration of communities of extended kin, on which African Americans had depended for many years for social, economic, and emotional support. Although ties were still maintained, they were disrupted and fragmented. Concurrently, many African Americans lost their pitifully small but stable incomes. And although opportunities increased for better jobs, especially through the Armed Forces, the spectre of unemployment was raised—something that was virtually unknown among rural African Americans before this.

These events also brought with them an increase in covert discrimination against African Americans. As one African American woman said who bucked all the odds and went to normal school in New Orleans in the 1920s:

What has changed is not the real opportunities for African Americans, which are still just as poor as ever, but the level of hypocrisy in Whites' attitudes. They say they are giving equal opportunity for jobs, but as soon as they know the color of your skin, they think of some excuse not to hire you. Nowadays the discrimination is much more insidious, more hidden. At least before, you knew where you stood.

Racism still runs deep, and perhaps even deeper because some Whites feel threatened by competition from African Americans. This may be what Emmelina meant when she said that times were better before World War II.

Changes in African American Family Structure Following World War II

It is from this perspective that one must view the changes that began to occur in African American families following World War II. Between 1940 and 1965—the time period during which most mothers of the adolescents interviewed in our larger-sample study were born—African American families started down one of three paths. One path was up the ladder of social and economic status, an avenue that was open particularly to the relatively small percentage of better-educated African American men and women who prior to mechanization had cultivated skills in nonagricultural domains. These skills and the personal characteristics that made their acquisition possible equipped these individuals to take advantage of newly available opportunities and to become the progenitors of present-day middle-class African American families, many of whom no longer live in the region. The move upward, however, was and is not without its own stressors, failures, and calamities.

A second path, taken by African American families who could not take immediate advantage of new opportunities, was to try as much as possible to maintain the status quo in terms of economic and social practices. Despite the growing stigma within the African American community attached to remaining on the plantation, those who did essentially bought time, holding steady long enough to allow a new generation to become educated, a work force to become more open to African Americans, and a society to become more accustomed to and comfortable with integration—trends that, in this region of the country, have perhaps taken longer than in some others but that are still clearly evident. In contrast, a third path, taken by those who were unable or unwilling to maintain the status quo or to take advantage of new opportunities, was to begin downhill toward what seems today to be an intractable "under-class" status. The rapid social, economic, and political changes in African Americans' environments, beginning with the Great Depression, thus amounted to what can be described as a "sink, swim, or tread water" state of affairs.

These three different directions and their relevance to the current-day social problem of adolescent pregnancy are illustrated in the next chapter by the situations of three women who, at the beginning of the ethnographic phase of our research, lived on three different plantations in the River Parish region. All were in their 20s when we met them; two had been unwed adolescent mothers, and the third eventually became an unwed (but not adolescent) mother. One, Aretha, is a third-generation member of a family that has succeeded in many respects in maintaining the status quo, a family that is functioning more or less like it was 100 years ago. The second, Yolanda, is from a family that is continuing a downwardly mobile slide toward under-class status begun in her parent's generation. The third, Rachel, is from a family whose components are in various stages of transition to middle-class status. In the following section, we present brief sketches of these women's lives; the forms that mating and childrearing practices take in their families; and the functions that the latter serve for individuals' survival, prosperity, and personal satisfaction.

3

Adolescent Pregnancy
In the River Parishes

Plantation communities for workers in the River Parish region are now much smaller in size than they used to be; plantation stores and many churches are gone, graveyards are overgrown, and wooden cabins and outhouses are deteriorating, gradually replaced by "modern" cinder block constructions with plumbing facilities. Houses that remain in these communities are occupied by men and women still employed on the plantations and their extended families and by former employees who are now too old or sick to work but have been allowed to remain in their houses rent free. As in the past, most of the residents of these communities are African American and poor. Although most of these residents recognize the stigma attached to living and working on a plantation and are aware that people in the towns look down at them, they choose to live there because at least seasonal jobs are available for the able-bodied men, living costs are lower, and children are safer.

THE MODERN-DAY TRADITIONAL FAMILY

One plantation community we visited in the ethnographic phase consisted of about 20 houses, most of which were occupied by members of a single extended family, which for the sake of identification we refer to as Martha's family (all names are fictitious). Martha was a 50-year-old great-grandmother to whom all other members of the family were related by blood or by marriage, legal or common-law. Most of her daughters, sons, grandchildren, nieces and nephews, siblings, and her current husband's extended family members lived within a stone's throw of each other near a bend in a dirt road winding through the sugarcane fields. Virtually all of the women in this extended family had their first children as unwed adolescents by men with whom they had no further contact and then entered into more stable, long-lasting, legal or common-law marriages. Most of the middle-age men who were healthy enough were employed to varying degrees as tractor drivers, mechanics, and general laborers on the plantation. Martha's extended family included not only those members residing on the plantation, but also those who lived in nearby towns and cities. Martha herself was one of 17 siblings, most of whom were still living in the vicinity. On a visit to Martha's church one Sunday, we learned that the preacher, most of the congregation, the deacons, and the choir were members of her extended family.

Martha's family constituted a well-functioning network of mutual support and exchange. A few months into the study, we had observed all manner of exchanges among members of this network, including those involving children, food, money, advice, care of the sick, social visits, emotional support, and services such as automobile repairs and transportation. In addition, we heard about members of the family coming to each other's rescue in lovers' quarrels, physical fights, employment matters, and a myriad of other day-to-day crises. When Martha backed her car into a big ditch during a daily driving summer rainstorm, for example, her daughter's common-law husband quickly appeared with three helpers and a truck to extricate Martha from the car and pull it out of the ditch, while another daughter appeared to drive Martha to where she had to go, leaving her own small children in the care of Martha's husband's niece. When the insurance lady showed up at Martha's house one day looking for money that Martha did not have, Martha sent her grandson to scavenge the community for spare change. When thugs mugged one of Martha's sons at a local drinking establishment, the favor was quickly returned by other members of Martha's family. When Martha's granddaughter's boyfriend was seen driving down the road with a rival girlfriend, various members of Martha's family made threatening anonymous phone calls to the rival girlfriend in hopes of scaring her away.

In Martha's modern-day traditional family, premarital sex and pregnancies were indirectly tied to economics. Having a first child out of wedlock by a relative stranger, often a much older man, was one among several strategies that this family used to ensure that new generations would remain within the bosom of the extended-family support network on which they relied so heavily for economic and other resources. The first child of virtually every woman in this family had been raised either jointly by mother and grandmother or greatgrandmother or by one of the latter alone, providing a source of continuing contact, shared interest, and concern between the adolescent girl and the older women in the family.

Although space does not permit a lengthy discussion of the other strategies used to ensure continued family unity, they included such things as Martha's deliberate and conscious "forgetting" of the existences and names of her sons' and grandsons' children by "outside women," children who might compete with her and other members of her extended family for her sons' and grandsons' attentions and loyalties; pressures on young adult men and women leading them to sabotage their chances for obtaining jobs that would require them to move away from the extended-family compound; and severe criticism of individuals who even contemplated leaving any of their worldly possessions to in-laws. All of these strategies, including the practice of having and rearing a first child out of wedlock in collaboration with mother or grandmother, pitted loyalties to blood relatives against loyalties to conjugal relatives and introduced tension between girlfriends and boyfriends, husbands and wives, and extended families whose members were intermingled in terms of both physical proximity and marital relationships. The common practice of men in Martha's extended family having numerous "outside" women with whom they had numerous children was both a reflection of and contributor to those tensions. One man, for example, openly boasted of having 12 outside women with whom he had an indeterminate number of children. Although these outside women and children never made an appearance or were mentioned by name, they were an underlying and continuing source of tension between him and the "inside" women in his life.

The Downwardly Mobile Family

On another plantation in the River Parishes was Yolanda, a 25-year-old woman currently living with Walter, a man much her senior who had worked on the plantation all his life as a domestic servant and gardener. Yolanda had 8 children between the ages of 1 month and 12 years, only the most recent by Walter and the rest by different fathers. The 10 of them occupied a sparsely furnished four-room cinder-block dwelling with indoor plumbing and air conditioning. When she and Walter broke up a few months after we met them, Walter arranged for Yolanda and the children to move rent free to an unoccupied wooden cabin about 200 yards away, consisting of three small rooms and a bathroom and lacking all amenities, including indoor plumbing. In this house, the 7 older children slept together in the bedroom and Yolanda, the baby, and whatever man was visiting her at the time slept together in the living room. According to Yolanda, in order to ensure privacy when a man was there, she simply locked the door to the children's bedroom. Only one other member of Yolanda's family of origin lived on this plantation—her twin sister Rowanda—and her extended family seemed fragmented and ineffective in providing needed services or support for its members. This fragmentation is illustrated by an anecdote told to us by Yolanda's next-door neighbor.

When we arrived for our tutoring session one day, Yolanda's children, who usually greeted us with enthusiastic shouts, were nowhere to be seen. According to Yolanda's neighbor, they were inside their house in the charge of Yolanda's oldest child, a 12-year-old son, with orders from their mother to let no one in and to stay there until her return. Yolanda was at the local police station, where she had been taken earlier that day under arrest. As the story went, Yolanda had asked her sister Rowanda to stay with her children one night while she went out drinking at a local bar. On the day Yolanda was arrested, Rowanda had confessed that she and Walter, Yolanda's boyfriend, had "messed with" each other that night. Yolanda and Rowanda then got into a fight during which Yolanda slashed Rowanda with a knife. In the midst of the violence, Yolanda's neighbor called the police. Yolanda later told us that she and Rowanda had a history of violent interactions ("We're not like puddin' and Jell-O, we're more like water and hot grease!") and that she, Yolanda, had been incarcerated several times for fighting. Rowanda, in turn, had her own troubles with the law. Not long before, the court had deemed her unfit to be a mother and ordered all of her children to be placed in foster homes.

In Yolanda's downwardly mobile family, premarital sex and pregnancies were directly tied to economics. In the 1950s, when machines were rapidly replacing the jobs held by African American men on the plantations, Yolanda's father was laid off, was forced to move his wife and children to town, became ill, and eventually died. During this chaotic time, according to Yolanda, the family was in serious crisis, with the father taking out his frustrations in drinking, philandering, and beating his wife and children. Mother, from Yolanda's descriptions, was generally ineffectual in coping with this overwhelming situation. At age 12, Yolanda could no longer stand the abuse and she left home; it was 3 days before her mother started looking for her. Later, when Yolanda was arrested for street-fighting as a juvenile, her mother told the police to keep her there because it might teach her a lesson. Not long after, Yolanda's mother went to visit relatives in California, and she has yet to return. Some indication of the rage that Yolanda felt growing up in this environment is reflected in an incident in which she threw her infant sibling into an unlit fireplace for crying too much.

When Yolanda left home, she moved in briefly with an older man, a "friend of the family," who supported her in exchange for sex. According to Yolanda, no self-respecting woman would agree to be a man's sexual partner unless she were receiving benefits from him, including money. The pattern, which she and other women in her family followed, was to have one steady man around at all times—husband or boyfriend, live-in or live-out—to provide a steady source of income. At one time, according to Yolanda, she received $500 a month from one of her live-out boyfriends primarily for being available for sex whenever he wanted it. Having a baby by a man, she said, gives a woman certain rights to that man's property, whether she is having sex with him or not. Whenever she needs something, she can ask her baby's daddy to help her out. Similarly, according to one of her boyfriends, having multiple girlfriends and children by many women is an advantage to a man whose employment situation is unsteady at best, because these relationships provide multiple home bases to which he can go without having to pay for rent or food. As he put it, "Why would a dog stay with one bitch if he can have all of them on the street?" In a sense, then, Yolanda has replaced her poorly functioning family support network with another consisting of loose associations of men and women, bound together by shared parenthood and sexual relationships, who share their meager financial and other resources.

The Upwardly Mobile Family

When we first began our study, Rachel was 20 years old, unmarried, and aspiring to become a student at a business school several miles away from the plantation on which she lived near her father, her grandmother Elvira, and her retarded uncle whom Elvira had cared for all his life. All three occupied Elvira's dilapidated plantation cabin in which, in Elvira's words, "I woke up and found myself" more than 80 years before. Rachel lived with an elderly "aunt" in an equally ramshackle structure nearby. Like Yolanda, Rachel appeared to lack close ties with an extended-family network. As the following anecdote illustrates, however, the ostensible reason for this fragmentation in Rachel's family had less to do with the inability of members to provide support services than with their unwillingness to do so.

One day when we were visiting Elvira on her birthday, Yvette, a middle-age granddaughter from the city, drove up in a new, bright-red sportscar. After Yvette and Elvira exchanged cordial words and we had introduced ourselves, Yvette informed us that she was a successful businesswoman and that her daughter, whose Corvette she was driving that day, was an actress. After a brief conversation, Yvette drove away. Elvira told us she hardly remembered what "that girl" looked like, it had been so long since she had come to visit. When we asked whether Yvette ever sent her money, Elvira laughed and said, "The day that girl sends me money will be the day I dies and goes to Heaven. When people goes and makes something out themselves, they always forgets about the ones they left behind!" As it turned out, many members of Elvira's extended family had gone and made something of themselves.

This anecdote points up a characteristic of the upwardly mobile family type that is crucial in understanding the difficulties that poor African Americans face in raising themselves to middle-class status. Although Rachel's extended family as a whole can be described as upwardly mobile, the different components of it are in varying stages of transition toward middle-class status, a condition that creates instability and stress for individuals in the family. Her father, it seems, had several liaisons with women, some resulting in legal marriages and others in common-law marriages. The extended families of at least two of these women were in the process of moving up the social and economic ladder. Yvette was an only child of one of these unions, and Rachel was an only child of the other. Rachel's father, however, had been unable to support his wives' ambitions for upward mobility, choosing instead to spend his money on alcohol and outside women. As a consequence, Rachel grew up in a family environment in which her mother's high expectations and pressures for performance were combined with an extreme scarcity of economic and other resources from her immediate or extended family.

Premarital sex and pregnancy, from Rachel's mother's upwardly mobile perspective, was an impediment to the all-important goal of improving the family's economic and social status. Indeed, when one of Rachel's half-sisters became pregnant as a teenager, her mother insisted that she marry the father of her child before giving birth. Although this marriage eventually ended in divorce, Rachel's half-sister and her husband had managed to complete their educations, find jobs, and buy their own home before divorcing. From Rachel's father's perspective, however, premarital sex and pregnancy was the norm in his "traditional" family of origin back on the plantation, to which he eventually returned.

The difficulties that these tensions within her family created for Rachel can be seen from the course of events that transpired in her life in adolescence and beyond. According to Rachel, her mother often communicated her high expectations and standards in ways that were intolerable, through excessively harsh physical discipline. Things came to a head between them when Rachel was 16 years old. Her mother, who worked two jobs during the day and one at night, tried to beat Rachel for not helping her lazy half-sister with her chores. Vowing that she would never strike her mother, Rachel packed her clothes and moved to the plantation to be near father and Elvira.

After high school, Rachel's plan was to enroll in college, still determined to continue her mother's relentless pursuit of upward mobility.

Although her tuition could be paid for by grants, there were many other expenses such as books, supplies, and transportation, and her salaries from her various part-time jobs were not enough to meet those expenses. She knew that her mother had saved up money over the years that she had used to help her older half-siblings attend college but for some reason was unwilling to lend money to Rachel. What angered Rachel the most was that her mother, who routinely lent her car to her other children (who in Rachel's eyes were lazy and worthless), refused to do the same for Rachel, whose own decrepit car frequently broke down, forcing her to miss work until she could find someone to fix it for free. Eventually, Rachel abandoned the hope of going to college, and now, 4 years later, has become an unmarried, unemployed mother.

Summary

Our observations of these three family contexts in the ethnographic phase of this study, therefore, led us to hypothesize that unwed adolescent pregnancies serve social and economic functions for both the modern-day traditional and downwardly mobile families but are seen as impediments to the attainment of goals in upwardly mobile families. These case illustrations also point to the tenuous nature of both the modern-day traditional and upwardly mobile forms of the African American family in an environment of economic scarcity. Although Martha's family has managed to maintain the extended-family support network, this has been possible because of the continued availability of jobs, however low-paying, for the men in the family. As agriculture in the region has become progressively more mechanized, the number of jobs like those held by men in Martha's family has continued to decrease, pointing to a bleak future for the modern-day traditional family in this area. And one can surmise that Rachel's mother's reluctance to help Rachel in her educational pursuits at least partly reflected her limited economic resources and the need to conserve them for her own continuing efforts to attain middle-class status.

SOME PSYCHOLOGICAL FUNCTIONS OF ADOLESCENT PREGNANCY

From the stories that women told us about their premarital mating and childbearing activities, it was clear that they thought about these activities, both consciously and unconsciously, in the contexts of their relationships with their parents, and particularly with their mothers. In retrospect, we were able to classify the relationships described to us by Martha and her granddaughter Aretha, and by Rachel and her mother, as *competitive* and the relationships described by Yolanda and her daughter Lynetta as representative of a category we later labeled *deprived*.

Two Competitive Triads

Although the scenarios painted by Aretha, Rachel, and their mothers differ in their specifics, in both there is an underlying theme in which mother (grandmother) comes across as the hostile heavy and the girl is allied with father (or fantasy of father) against mother. Father comes to the girl's rescue in reality or in fantasy when mother becomes threatening.

Aretha. Aretha became pregnant as an unwed adolescent in the midst of an intense battle with Martha, her grandmother, that started when Aretha began to menstruate. In Martha's account of the events leading up to Aretha's pregnancy, she sat right down with Aretha and told her the same thing her Mama had told her: "Now Aretha, you got to watch them young boys out there nowadays because they'll try to entice you to go to bed with them, and the first thing you know, you're gonna pop up pregnant, and you ain't gonna be able to take care of no baby. You're too young to be taking care of a baby, and I'm too old to be trying to take care of babies." But, Martha lamented, "It didn't do no good, she still pop up pregnant."

As soon as Aretha started menstruating, Martha began the ritual of maintaining watch over Aretha's periods and activities, imposing strict curfews and restrictions on her contacts with boys and trying to drive away anyone who risked visiting Aretha on the plantation. Although boys would try to come by the house to talk to Aretha, Martha would chase them all away before they even had a chance to sit down on the porch. Martha said, "Aretha's older sisters all popped up pregnant, and I didn't want that for her." However, one particularly persistent boy, who lived one field down from Martha, started walking down the levee and would pass right behind Martha's backyard. When Aretha would see him walking up there, she would say, "Mama, I can't stand that little boy walking up there on that levee, I can't stand that little boy." After a while, Martha told Aretha, "Don't keep saying that. You don't know that boy. You can't say you don't like that little boy. Don't say that, you might end up going with that child." So, one day the boy came down the levee and asked Martha, "Where your granddaughter is? I like your granddaughter!" Martha then replied, "Oh, she at home. But please don't go over there and say nothing to her, because she gonna curse you, she gonna curse your name." And he used to tell Martha, "That's gonna be my girlfriend right there." "And sure enough," said Martha, "that's when he started talking to Aretha." And that's when Martha started taking Aretha for repeated examinations for suspected but nonexistent pregnancies at the health clinic. Aretha, in the meantime, played the innocent victim who either had no interest in going out or was forcibly "stuck under my grandmother," feeling unjustly maligned because "I wasn't doin' nothing."

When Martha discovered that Aretha was pregnant, her fury was at a peak; she was "shocked and humiliated," and Aretha cowered in fear. But because "what's done is done," both Martha and Aretha agreed to go ahead and have the baby. Martha's fury abated gradually over the remaining months of Aretha's pregnancy and ended with Martha and Aretha eagerly awaiting the baby's arrival. When the baby was born, Martha insisted that Aretha give her the baby to raise, not marry the baby's father, and continue living at home with her, but Aretha resisted these pressures and took the opposite course. According to Aretha, she became pregnant in the first place to "escape Martha's clutches" and to get away from the constant battles that took place between Martha and her alcoholic husband, Robert—a difficult task given Martha's constant vigilance. Aretha's vehicle of escape, interestingly, was her own father, who had somehow come back into her life the previous year after a lifetime of absence. Despite having seen her father only once before this, when she and her mother had been out driving one day, Aretha had an intense fantasy relationship with him as a child, always imagining that he would come by in his truck and take her away from her mean grandmother and stepfather. Aretha, in fact, became pregnant in her father's house while "housesitting." Her boyfriend, being the son of one of Martha's good friends with whom she had a weekly game of Pokeno, was "the only boy I knew who wasn't afraid of Martha." According to Aretha, she would never give one of her babies to Martha to raise; these were her babies, although she did not mind if the children spent most of every day at Martha's. With each of Aretha's successive pregnancies, the battle for possession of her babies continued.

Rachel. Rachel's mother described Rachel as a child who would never listen, who would do all kinds of "dumb" things around the house, who would always "jump on my back," and who got on her nerves. No matter when she told Rachel to be home or what she told her to do, Rachel always ended up somewhere else doing something else. The only way her mother could keep her from doing those things was to "always be running after her" or to "give her a few whacks" with a switch or whatever was at hand. For example, one night when Rachel was about 14, Rachel's mother let Rachel go to a school pageant in the charge of her "best cousin" Lionel. About 10:00, Lionel came home without Rachel, saying that when it came time to leave, Rachel was nowhere to be found. Rachel's mother was beside herself with worry. She said to her own mama, "My daughter is out there in that world, and I'm going to find her. I was wondering if she be by herself, nervous as I don't know what! So I went back and forth to her school two times with tears flowing down my eyes. So I come back the second time, and I look down this little alley going towards this way, and I looked, and I saw girls going down the alley. So I went running over there to see if she was with them. I didn't see her. So I come back towards Winn-Dixie, and when I come back, she was coming. I said 'Girl, get yourself over here!' She said, 'Mama, you making me ashamed.' I said, 'I don't care. Get over here! You're not going nowhere no more.' She said, 'Mama, shut up all that hollering.' I said, 'I ain't shutting up nothing cause you ain't got no business out there by yourself like this. And these little boys out here be crazy and drunk, and this and that and the other. And you out there!' . . . And after that, she didn't ask no more to go out with friends."

Rachel had a very different view of her life with mother. She initially described her mother as a person who was indispensable in teaching her how to be a woman. She remembered back when her mother showed her how to cook, to clean house, to iron, and to perform other domestic chores. She was especially grateful to her mother, and later to her grandmother, for explaining to her about "female" things: sex, pregnancy, menstruation, and men. She felt she owed her mother the utmost respect and devotion, and she felt she should sacrifice her own needs for her mother's sake, even though her mother gave her little in return.

As her story continued, less positive aspects of Rachel's relationship with her mother began to emerge. Rachel's troubles with her mother began, she felt, at the age of 6 when her parents divorced. Until that time, she had been her father's favorite, and he had always intervened on her behalf when problems arose between them. When her father and mother would become engaged in violent physical fights over his activities with other women, Rachel would intervene physically on behalf of her father. When her parents divorced, her father left home and moved in with his mother and retarded brother on the plantation, leaving Rachel at the mercy of her mother's beatings. According to Rachel, her mother took revenge and began mistreating her. Resentment that Rachel had allied herself with her father was, according to Rachel, the real reason why her mother severely restricted her activities and disciplined her excessively and unfairly. When she could no longer stand this treatment, Rachel turned again to her father and the safe haven of the plantation.

A Deprived Dyad

Lynetta, Yolanda's daughter who was 11 when our study began and 16 when she gave birth to her first child as an unwed mother, also became pregnant in the context of an intense battle with Yolanda that had much the same flavor as that between Martha and Aretha. According to Yolanda, when Lynetta did not get her way, she would throw temper tantrums: "Once she and her older brother got into something, and I mean, she was really terrible then. Because she threw a knife at him, and it stuck right up in his arm. And I mean, he had to have stitches. It was bad. And there were lots of other times, like when she had a boyfriend, and I thought she was going overboard, getting too deep in it, and I told her about him and another girl. And oh, she cried. She went in her room and cried and she cried and she cried. And um, she took some pills, some aspirin or something. And, you know, she was lying in her bed, and I went to go see about her. And I saw that she had the bottle on her dresser, and it was open . . . You know it was like, it was open for everybody to see."

After Lynetta became pregnant, her story diverged from Aretha's. When Yolanda discovered that Lynetta was pregnant, she responded violently and threw her out of the house. Lynetta then went to live with her boyfriend. Six weeks after the baby was born, it died while spending the night in bed with Yolanda and her boyfriend, officially from Sudden Infant Death Syndrome.

In separate interviews when Lynetta was about 12, she and Yolanda talked about their feelings about mothers and motherhood. To paraphrase them, Yolanda stated that when she was young she had wanted to be a child therapist, a marriage counselor, or a lawyer, but things changed after she met her boyfriend. She still might want to do those things, but she feels it is better to just take care of her children. If everybody would decide the way she did, to stay home and care for their children, the world would be a different place. According to Yolanda, "All children be bad, they can't be good. Even infants is bad." Her mother taught her mothering skills because she loved her. "She had to have loved me if she took care of me and I was that bad." Mothers must really love their children if they go through all the trouble of putting up with them. People are closer to their mothers than to their fathers because mothers went through all that "sweat and pain" to have children: "When your father dies, you forget about him in a couple of months, but when your mother dies, you always miss her." When Yolanda was a little girl, "I used to tell my doll, I'm gonna kill you." When little children made noise, "I thought I wanted to kill them. But when I got older, all that changed. Now, I'm the best mother, because my children need me and I need them. I'd be willing to die for my children because Christ died for us, so I'd be willing to die for my children." During this one conversation, Yolanda spontaneously brought up the subject of child abuse six times. She recounted an incident in which her second daughter burned herself badly as a 2-year-old. When she took the child to the hospital, she could tell what the nurse was thinking, and Yolanda told her, "If you don't stop thinking that, I don't know what I'm gonna do to you." According to Yolanda, it's acceptable to spank your children, but there is no need to "beat them into the grave." Her own mother did not spank her, she just sat down and talked about what to do right and wrong. Lynetta said that she sometimes gets in fights with other girls at school because they tease her about her mother. She said, "If people at school talked about my Dad, I wouldn't do nothing. If they talked about my Mama, I would want to kill them. Your mama did all the hard work in bringing you into this world. She could die with you." Lynetta did not think she wanted to be a mother because she did not think that adults want to be adults: "They're wishing they were a child." However, she knew that her "Mom and Dad really love taking care of me." When she grows up, she wants to "give my mom something to remember me by." It occurred to us at the time that one very valuable gift that poor African American adolescent girls give to their mothers in this community is a baby.

In contrast to Rachel's and Aretha's stories, these two interviews with Yolanda and Lynetta stress the dyadic relationship between mother and daughter, with father taking an explicitly secondary role. In both interviews, a predominant underlying theme includes the feelings of deprivation, yearning, and rage conveyed by both women about their relationships with mother, combined with an obvious but only partially successful attempt to deny these feelings. Both women's ambivalent feelings regarding their relationships with their own mothers, moreover, are reflected in their feelings about their real or anticipated relationships with their own children. Particularly striking in these interviews is the strength of Lynetta's identification with Yolanda's unconscious conflicts.

Summary

Thus, it seemed from our conversations with women in Martha's traditional family and in Yolanda's downwardly mobile family that there was a part of these women that had wanted to become pregnant in adolescence and a part of them that had not. The part that had wanted to become pregnant was manifested by their actions. According to their own stories, these women had deliberately and voluntarily put themselves in situations where the likelihood of the occurrence of sexual intercourse was high. All had voluntarily consented to intercourse. All had knowledge that sexual intercourse can lead to pregnancy. None had used any form of protection against pregnancy, although for the younger women in particular, such measures were not only known to them and accessible but had been stressed by their mothers.

The part of them that had not wanted to become pregnant was manifested by the stories they constructed to explain their actions to themselves and to others. These explanations had the quality of post hoc rationalizations of behavior that they themselves did not truly understand, of intentions they did not want to acknowledge to themselves or to us. These women described their deliberate and voluntary acts as if they had "just happened," as if they had just found themselves in situations where sexual intercourse was inevitable, without any prior thought or planning. We thought it implausible that these acts could have "just happened," particularly in the light of what was described as very active efforts on the parts of their mothers to prevent such occurrences and in light of the girls' own statements that they were "doin' nothing" and did not wish to become pregnant. These explanations were also inconsistent with their explicit verbalizations regarding the adverse consequences of an adolescent pregnancy with respect to educational and economic opportunities and inconsistent with what we knew about the planful, intelligent, and informed manner in which they conducted the rest of their lives.

Similar contradiction and conflict was evident with respect to some mothers' wishes about their daughters' (granddaughters') sexual activity and pregnancies. Again, the part of them that seemed to want their daughters to become sexually active and pregnant was manifested by their actions, which served to engineer and direct the unfolding of the sequence of events leading to pregnancy, the initial hostile reaction to the pregnancy followed by eventual acceptance, and the ultimate disposition of the baby's care in the hands of the mother or mother–daughter duo. The part of them that did not want their daughters to become pregnant was manifested by the surface meaning of their actions and verbal statements to their daughters about sexual activity and pregnancy, by their statements to us about their feelings of shame and disappointment about their daughters' pregnancies, and by their clear understanding that adolescent pregnancy can interfere with a girl's opportunity to "raise herself up" out of poverty. These mothers' explanations for these events had the same quality of post hoc rationalization as the girls' explanations: "It just happened"; "There was nothing I could do," "If a girl wants to get pregnant, there's nothing anybody can do about it"; "Now that the baby is here, there's nothing I can do but love it."

An Informal Theory of Adolescent Pregnancy

Having arrived at the conclusion that unwed adolescents' pregnancies are both consciously unintended and unconsciously intended, I set about the task of trying to understand the system that integrates these two contradictory aspects of people's minds and lives. The system I envisioned consisted of sociocultural–historical and individual psychological pieces, relations among these pieces, and dynamic forces that operate to hold the system together despite external and internal pressures to the contrary. In the remainder of this chapter, I briefly review the pieces as I conceptualized them in general form at the end of the ethnographic phase.

Evolutionary Conservatism

One piece in the adolescent pregnancy system was suggested by the historical review in chapter 2, which indicated that adolescent pregnancy in the African American population has been adapted over time to a variety of specific uses, all of which have been in the service of the general, overarching goal of maintaining networks. Throughout history, adolescent pregnancies and births have facilitated networking by providing manpower for the protection of tribes and womanpower for the continued production of manpower, by enticing slave owners to keep families together, by consolidating networks of support and exchange in the face of oppression and economic scarcity, or by developing extra-kin networks of support and exchange to replace the extended-family network. These changes in the specific ways that adolescent pregnancy has been used to support networking, in turn, reflect historical changes in the larger sociocultural contexts of people's lives from precolonial times to the present day. The perpetuation of the adolescent pregnancy behavior pattern in this population despite changing times and contexts illustrates what others (e.g., Bates, Benigni, Bretherton, Camaioni, & Volterra, 1979) have suggested is a conservative trend in evolution. When the need for specialized functions arises, old structures and customs serving old purposes are not jettisoned, but rather kept, fine-tuned, and reused for the new purposes.

Multiple Contexts

A second conservative force motivating the perpetuation of the adolescent pregnancy system is its overdetermined nature. In this regard, LeVine (1982) had this to say:

Concretely, the individual in his pattern of behavior has at least two "reasons" for his behavior; It allows him satisfaction of private motives and it accords with what is socially prescribed. In addition, it may well be consistent with the personal standards he internalized through the deliberate socialization by his parents, and it is likely to have an ideological justification in a religious or ethical doctrine. These diverse sources converge in providing support for his pattern of behavior. Though each factor might seem to constitute an adequate explanation in itself, and in the case of a particular individual not all factors are necessarily involved, all contributed to the history of the pattern and all are involved in its maintenance as a population characteristic rather than an idiosyncrasy. Its overdetermined nature, by diversifying the grounds for its social acceptability and popular appeal and by a reinforcing consistency in influencing the individual, contributes greatly to its stability as a pattern of psychosocial adaptation. (p. 165)

Observations in the ethnographic phase suggested that reasons for adolescent sexual behavior of whatever form occur at conscious and unconscious levels within individuals' minds; at implicit and explicit levels of discourse in the sociocultural environment; in multiple family environment contexts; in the context of multiple, culturally constituted success schemata; in the contexts of multiple representations of attachment relationships within the mother–daughter dyad; and in the context of multiple representational schemes on the parts of mothers with regard to daughters' adolescent sexual activities. Adolescent sexual activity and pregnancy, therefore, is highly overdetermined.

Family Environment Contexts

A piece of the adolescent pregnancy system discovered in the ethnographic phase was that networking functions of adolescent pregnancy among poor, African American women differ as a function of family environment context; networking functions are crucial for survival in downwardly mobile and traditional families, but can interfere with goals in upwardly mobile families. In downwardly mobile environments, poorly functioning, extended-kin support networks are supplemented or replaced by extra-kin networks of unmarried men and women, bound together in part by shared parenthood and sexual relationships. Women receive financial and other kinds of support from the several fathers or prospective fathers of their children, whereas men receive the same from the several mothers or prospective mothers of their children. In traditional family environments, relatively better functioning extended-kin networks are maintained and strengthened by mothers' and adolescent daughters' common bond with and shared goal of raising first-born (and perhaps later-born) children conceived out of wedlock. In contrast, upwardly mobile families avoid and discourage networking among extended kin that interferes with the superordinate goal of improving social and economic status. Thus, adolescent pregnancy is not a uniform phenomenon in this sociocultural milieu, but has multiple functions that are tied to variations in the structural and networking characteristics of family environments.

Cultural Success Schemas

Differences in the implicit functions served by adolescent pregnancy in different family environments are paralleled by differences in culturally constituted schemas of success and survival. Women and men in all three family environments explicitly represent "success" in terms of a stereotypical middle-class family existence. Intermediate points along the road to attaining this goal include graduating from high school and college, the getting and keeping of jobs, finding a steady mate, buying a house, and having children when it is economically feasible to support them. In all three family environments, people consciously aspire to such an existence and are aware that having babies out of wedlock in adolescence can make this goal harder to attain.

However, some people behaved, talked, and felt in ways that suggested a competing, less conscious, culturally constituted cognitive success (survival) schema. Success in this schema consists not of attaining middle-class status but of forging the kinds of networks that ensure survival in a socioeconomic environment fraught with perceived insurmountable obstacles to the attainment of middle-class status. Points along the way to achieving this goal include unwed adolescents' pregnancies among others aimed at keeping productive individuals emotionally, financially, and socially tied to the extended-kin or extra-kin network.

Mother–Daughter Relationships

A further theme could be inferred from the stories women told us about their premarital and childbearing activities. It was clear that women thought about these activities, both consciously and unconsciously, in the context of their relationships with parents, and especially with mothers. In retrospect, some of these stories could be classified as reflecting competitive representations and others as reflecting deprived representations. A third category, termed *mature,* was later identified in the larger-sample interview phase. As noted with regard to culturally constituted success schemas, some aspects of these schemas were conscious and others were less so. Most notably, in the deprived relationship context, women were conscious of their wishes to be good mothers and to receive good mothering or fathering, and they were unconscious of the less acceptable and competing wishes to harm or abandon their children, to retaliate against their mothers or fathers for felt rejections or injuries, and to give mother a gift to forestall further rejections or to make up for unacceptable wishes to retaliate. In the competitive relationship context, women were conscious of their desires to escape from the clutches of their presumably hostile and demanding mothers but unconscious of the wishes to achieve victory over mothers vis-à-vis relationships with father and to atone for the latter. In both relationship contexts, the anticipation of conceiving and bearing a child played an important role in women's unconscious representations of these wishes.

Mothers' Explicit and Implicit Messages

Another dynamic identified in the ethnographic phase was the dual roles played by mothers in the adolescent pregnancy system—one of creating social and emotional contexts for daughter's psychological development and the other of communicating implicit and explicit messages about the desirability or undesirability of daughter's entrance into puberty, dating, and sexual activities with boys; use of contraceptives; and pregnancy. Explicit messages were communicated verbally through the content of mothers' statements about boys, sex, birth control devices, rules, attributions about daughters' activities and intentions, and the like. Implicit messages were communicated from mothers to daughters through primarily nonverbal means. These included the degree of consistency between mothers' words, deeds, and emotional reactions; the timing of mothers' communications to daughters in relation to daughters' opportunities for dating and sexual activities; and the degree to which mothers were emotionally engaged with daughters in matters having to do with daughters' entrances into puberty, sexuality, and pregnancy, including the emotional intensities of mothers' emotional responses to daughters' actual or presumed dating and sexual activities. Mothers' implicit messages reflect their own unconscious representations of what is required for survival and success in their particular family environments as well as their own mostly unconscious representations of what is desired in the context of their relationships with daughters. Conflicting messages from mothers derive from conflicts within the cultural milieu and within themselves regarding the desirability of the adolescent pregnancy outcome.

4

Finding Patterns and Meanings Through Qualitative and Quantitative Methods

A helpful metaphor in describing the evolution of a complex system is a symphony, a dynamic creation in which principal themes and subthemes are played and replayed, developed and redeveloped, differentiated and integrated with varying degrees of dissonance or consonance in ever-changing contexts until they come to some final resolution. In the ethnographic phase of this project, some themes of the adolescent pregnancy symphony as it plays out in this particular population of poor African Americans came through loud and clear. Moreover, these themes and some of their variations, which were described at the end of the previous chapter, could be made to fit together in ways that make intuitive sense, in ways that are pleasing to the ear.

To carry the symphony metaphor further, questions remain as to how much of the total work was actually heard during that phase of the study, how much of what was heard is theme and how much is variation, how much is central to the structural unity and development of the composition versus an interesting digression away from it, and how much the fit inferred among themes in that phase of the research is representative of the many ways these themes in fact do fit together in this population. Whereas the ethnographic method of participant observation with small numbers of individual families is well suited for the discovery of themes and a description of how they fit together in particular contexts (e.g., particular individuals, particular families; i.e., the close-up view), it is less well-suited as a method for discovering the universe of themes, variations, and ways in which themes weave together in the symphony as a whole (i.e., the broader view). What was needed following the ethnographic phase, therefore, was a methodology that could separate out the multiple themes from particular contexts in order to identify the many and complex ways in which they are developed, integrated, and resolved.

In the second phase of the research, therefore, interviews were conducted with a larger sample of poor African American teenage girls and their mothers, focused in particular on those content domains that emerged as potentially relevant to adolescent pregnancy in the ethnographic phase—that is, mothers' and adolescent daughters' representations of their personal relationships, of their family environments, and of daughters' adolescent sexuality and mothers' and daughters' explicit and implicit methods of communicating to each other the content of these representations. Both quantitative and qualitative data analysis procedures were used to extract themes and to examine their interrelations. In effect, the goals of this phase were to understand (a) in what ways mothers' and daughters' personal and cultural representations corresponded or did not correspond to those of women in the ethnographic study and (b) how personal and cultural representations work together in the adolescent pregnancy system.

From a methodological standpoint, the task of figuring out what people mean from their responses to interview questions poses a special challenge, inasmuch as the people themselves do not entirely know what they mean. Meanings inherent in personal or cultural representations are partly hidden from the conscious awareness of the individuals who think them. Meanings inherent in conscious representations of relationships, of selves, of desirable outcomes, of motives, of paths to success and security, and the like may often be quite different if not opposite from those inherent in unconscious representations. Thus, if the purpose of a study is to identify both unconscious and conscious implicit and explicit meanings, it is not enough to ask people to describe their perspectives or to explain their behavior because they themselves are not fully aware of the forces in the culture or within themselves that motivate them one way or the other.

Throughout this research, a consistent strategy was used to identify and understand meanings that centered around the identification and interpretation of observable, repetitive patterns in people's narratives. Consistent patterns are reflections of something meaningful going on in the mind of an individual or a group that merit further study. Although patterns always make sense after their underlying meanings are known, patterns in themselves are never sufficient to infer these underlying meanings because correspondences between patterns and meanings are imperfect; the same essential meaning can be reflected by different patterns, and the same pattern may mean different things in different contexts. From a methodological standpoint, then, one difficulty is figuring out which of several possible patterns discernable in a stream of data best captures the essence of meanings hidden in the data; another is figuring out how to use patterns discernable in the data to elucidate the hidden meanings they reflect. As is evident from the circularity implied by these two challenges, the two processes of identifying patterns and the meanings they represent must proceed apace.

In the second or larger-sample phase of this study, the strategy of discerning meanings from patterns began with the structuring of interview situations such that observable responses (emotional, verbal, behavioral) of mothers and daughters would likely be influenced by the underlying phenomena of interest. Two interview situations in particular—the Adult Attachment Interview (AAI) (George et al., 1985), administered to mother and daughter individually in modified forms, and a joint-interview session with mother and daughter about problematic relationship issues—generated observable responses relevant to both personal and cultural constructs.

Then, from observable responses relevant to a given theme, a smaller number of composite variables was constructed representing latent constituent components of the underlying construct. In some cases, we knew ahead of time which responses to put together in these composite variables; in others, we used principal components factor analysis to identify composite variables. Ultimately, this step in the process contributed to both the finding of patterns and the understanding of their meanings. Patterns are more easily discernable in a smaller than a larger data set; meanings are more readily interpretable from a combination of related responses than from a single response.

The next step was to search for patterns in individuals' scores across these constituent variables. Our method of searching for patterns was to use cluster analysis, a statistical procedure that is not only blind to the meaning of the patterns it finds but is influenced by such vagaries as the number of clusters requested and the order in which constituent variables are entered. To choose among different possible configurations of patterns resulting from these analyses, we relied most heavily on the criterion of meaningfulness. Sets of patterns were chosen that made sense in relation to prior qualitative analyses of ethnographic and interview material. Sets of patterns consistent with these qualitative referents were selected as indicators of the underlying construct if patterns in the set were reliably distinguishable one from the other and if each pattern in the set was associated with sufficiently large numbers of mothers or daughters to allow for further data analysis.

The final step in the process complemented the previous ones by using observed interrelations among figurative patterns to further elucidate the meanings of the underlying constructs. Interrelations among sets of patterns create a contextual framework within which individual pieces take on more meaning than in isolation. Knowing whether and how personal and cultural representations relate to family environments, for example, yields a deeper understanding of what those family environments are about than one would have from descriptions of family environments alone. In these ways, we met the challenges of identifying patterns and their hidden meanings in the larger-sample interview phase by trading back and forth between one and the other to find both of them.

In the remainder of this chapter, I describe the particulars of the individuals included in the larger sample and of the measures used to obtain information about cultural and personal representational themes and variations.

The Study

Participants

The people interviewed in the larger-sample phase of the research were 87 African American teenage girls ranging in age from 14 to 19 years and the central maternal figures (hereafter referred to as *mothers*) who raised them. Of these, 2 were grandmothers, 3 were aunts, one was a stepmother, one was an adoptive mother, and 80 were biological mothers of the teens. Daughters were recruited through local high schools and health clinics in the region and were selected for the study on the basis of (a) their pregnancy status, with an attempt made to include approximately equal numbers of teens who had and had not become pregnant by the time of the interview; (b) the family's income level, with only those included who were eligible for the free school-lunch program as determined by federal poverty guidelines (Social Security Bulletin, 1989); and (c) the willingness of both the teen and her mother to participate.[1]

---

[1] When mother and teen arrived at the interview site, the interviewer restated the purpose of the study and read aloud the contents of a consent form. A copy of the form is shown in Appendix E. Mother and teen were asked if they understood the purpose and requirements of the study and if they would voluntarily agree to participate. Those who agreed (and all did) were asked to sign the form. Information regarding the ages of the mother and teen, current family composition, employment history, and family income was then gathered on an intake form. At the end of the interview sessions, both mother and teen were paid $25 for their participation.

The final sample included 45 ever-pregnant teens (mean age = 16.86 years, SD = 1.65), 42 never-pregnant teens (mean age = 16.02 years, SD = 1.28), and their 87 mothers (mean age = 40.94 years, SD = 7.5). Of these 87 mothers, 51 had been pregnant as adolescents. For the total sample of 87 dyads, the mean annual combined income for all occupants of a household was $11,327, the mean number of occupants per household was 5.16, and the mean income per occupant was $2,387. Virtually all teens were attending high school at the time of our interviews. Mean number of years of education for mothers was 8.92.

For purposes of examining historical trends in our data, we subsequently divided the mothers into two cohorts: those older than the mean who were born between the late 1930s and 1952 and those younger than the mean who were born later than 1952.[2] In the older mother cohort, 32% had given birth to a child as a teenager, compared to 80% in the younger mother cohort. Seventy percent of older mothers who had given birth as an unwed teenager married within a year of their first birth, compared to 57% of the younger mothers and 0% of the teens in the same category.

The Procedure

In this study, the AAI was used for three purposes. The first was to assess mothers' and daughters' representations of their attachment relationships. The second was to obtain information about participants' representations of their past and present family environments, obtained from "warm-up" questions already included in the beginning of the interview. The third was to assess participants' beliefs about, knowledge of, attitudes about, and practices of sex, pregnancy, and birth control obtained from questions that our research group added at the end of the interview.[3,4]

In the first part of each session, one interviewer administered the AAI to the mother and a second interviewer administered the AAI to the teen. Two forms of the AAI were given to the mother in counterbalanced order. One (the mother–mother interview) focused on her representations of her past and current primary attachment relationships with parents and siblings. The other (the mother–teen interview) focused on mother's representations of her daughter's past and current relationships with herself and with daughter's father. Questions in the daughter's interview (the teen interview) were identical to those in the mother–mother interview; that is, they focused on the respondent's past and current primary attachment relationships. All AAIs were audiotaped and later transcribed verbatim. Transcriptions included not only the words spoken by interviewer and interviewee, but the nuances of how they were spoken (e.g., timing, inflection, emphasis, feeling).

The mother and her daughter were brought together after the administration of the AAI for 10 to 20 min and questioned about problematic areas of their current relationship. These joint interviews were videotaped.

---

[2] Thirty-eight mothers were older than the mean (mean age = 47.53 years, *SD* = 6.5), and 49 were younger than the mean (mean age = 35.84 years, *SD* = 2.6).

[3] Procedures for coding responses to questions about sex, pregnancy, and birth control are described in Appendix B, section B (-1-b). Procedures for coding responses to questions about family environments are described in Appendix B, section A (-1-a).

[4] To prepare for the administration of the AAI in this study, Anne L. Dean and one collaborator, Mary Malik, were trained at a workshop conducted by Roger Kobak in May 1989.

The AAI

The interview. The AAI (George et al., 1985) is a structured series of questions and probes focusing on adolescents' or adults' early attachment relationships and experiences. The task confronting the interviewee is to access, organize, express, reflect on, and evaluate early memories, thoughts, and feelings relevant to attachment. Individual presentations vary in the degree to which they can be characterized as coherent or incoherent, manifested by implicit adherence or lack thereof to four discourse maxims identified by Grice (1975): "quality (be truthful and have evidence for what you say); quantity (be succinct yet complete); relation (be relevant or perspicacious); and manner (be clear and orderly)" (Main, 1995, p. 438). An individual's mode of discourse on the AAI has been variously deemed reflective of his or her "state of mind," "quality of thought," or "internal working model" about attachment relationships. In this book, from now on, we use the phrase *quality of thought* to refer to respondents' discourse modes on the AAI.

An important characteristic of the AAI is its goal to surprise the unconscious by catching the respondents off guard (George et al., 1985). The first set of questions focusing on factual aspects of the early family situation (family composition, residence patterns, parents' occupational history, and extended kin) is intended to put the respondents at ease. The next request from the interviewer, "I'd like you to try to describe your relationship with your parents as a young child," changes the subject without warning and is intended to activate both the respondents' unconscious conflicts with regard to these relationships and their habitual cognitive modes of processing these conflicts. Subsequent interview requests continue the focus on attachment issues, alternately probing for general and specific descriptions of the respondents' childhood and current attachment relationships. Interviewees are asked to supply five adjectives[5] describing their relationship with mother during childhood and another five describing their early relationship with father; they are then asked for specific memories that exemplify those adjectival descriptions. Other questions ask about (a) whether the interviewees felt closer to mother or father and why and (b) experiences of rejection, loss, and threatening or abusive behavior by parents. Finally, questions are included that ask for evaluations and reflections about the effects of these experiences on the interviewees' development and subsequent relationships.

Four classifications derived by Main and her colleagues for individual respondents on the AAI are the secure, the dismissing, the preoccu-

---

[5] Some interviewees in this study were unsure as to the meaning of the term *adjective*, so we substituted the term *word*.

pied, and the unresolved/disorganized. These classifications are counterparts respectively of the secure, insecure–avoidant, insecure–ambivalent/resistant, and disorganized categories of infant behavior exhibited in the Strange Situation (Ainsworth, Blehar, Waters, & Wall, 1979; Main & Soloman, 1986). In addition, a subset of interviews fall into the "cannot classify" category if the respondent alternates between discourse modes or if the quality of incoherence manifested does not correspond to any of the predetermined classifications (Main, 1995).[6]

The secure individual, to paraphrase Main's (1995) description, presents and evaluates memories of attachment experiences coherently, consistently, clearly, and succinctly, and she is relevant in what she chooses to present. The secure individual can shift flexibly between questions and the memories called upon; is ready to reexamine past relationships, feelings, and statements during the interview (a quality termed *metacognitive monitoring* by Main); and is ready to admit that her memories are influenced by her own subjective viewpoint.

Two "organized" insecure classifications are the dismissing and the preoccupied. Dismissing individuals minimize the importance of attachment-related experiences. Responses to questions appear superficially collaborative, but internal inconsistences and contradictions in their responses "render them apparently untruthful" (Main, 1995, p. 440). Dismissing individuals claim frequently not to remember and tend to cut the interviewer short with brief replies or insistence on lack of memory. This pattern, Main suggested, thus constitutes "a kind of resistance to the task" (p. 440).

Preoccupied individuals maintain an "excessive, confused and either angry or passive preoccupation with attachment figures or attachment-related events, as shown in violations of manner, relevance and quantity" (p. 441)—a style that Main suggested is not fully conscious. As for the dismissing pattern, said Main, preoccupation also represents a kind of resistance to the interview process in that it often overwhelms the interviewer, making it difficult to conduct the interview completely and efficiently.

The unresolved/disorganized interview is characterized by mental disorganization and disorientation, identified as lapses in the monitoring of

---

[6] Attachment classifications resulting from the AAI have been shown to be stable over 2-month (Bakersmans-Kranenburg & van Ilzendoorn, 1993), 3-month (Sagi et al., 1994) and 12-month (Benoit & Parker, 1994) periods and to have concurrent (e.g., Crowell & Feldman, 1988; Grossman, Fremmer-Bombik, Rudolph, & Grossman, 1988; Kobak & Sceery, 1988; Rice, 1991; van Ilzendoorn & Kroonenberg, 1988), predictive (Benoit & Parker, 1994; Benoit, Vidovic, & Roman, 1991; Fonagy, Steele, & Steele, 1991, in press; Radojevic, 1992; van Ilzendoorn, 1995; van Ilzendoorn & Kroonenberg, 1988; Ward & Carlson, 1991, 1995), and discriminant (Bakersmans-Kranenburg & van Ilzendoorn, 1993; Sagi et al., 1994; Waters et al., 1993) validities.

reasoning or discourse, especially during discussions of potentially traumatic events such as about loss, death, or sexual abuse (Main, 1995). Respondents classified as unresolved/disorganized are always also placed in a second best fitting category (secure, preoccupied, or dismissing).

From a theoretical vantage point, classifications on the AAI have been said to reflect an individual's internal working model of attachment relationships (Bowlby, 1973; Bretherton, 1985, 1990, 1991; Main, 1995; Main et al., 1985). As phrased by Main et al. (1985), internal working models are

> a set of conscious and/or unconscious rules for the organization of information relevant to attachment and for obtaining access to that information, that is, to information regarding attachment-related experiences, feelings and ideations. . . . Secure versus the various types of insecure attachment organizations can best be understood as terms referring to particular types of internal working models of relationships, models that direct not only feelings and behavior but also attention, memory and cognition, insofar as these relate directly or indirectly to attachment. Individual differences in these internal working models will therefore be related not only to individual differences in patterns of nonverbal behavior but also to patterns of language and structures of mind. (p. 67)

More recently, Main (1995) speculated that violations of discourse maxims on the AAI may have the goal of maintaining a dismissing or preoccupied attentional/representational state that is used by the individual to maintain self-organization and reduce anxiety in the face of memories of a rejecting or inconsistently available parent. These states have their origins in infancy in the behavioral strategies that the infant used to maintain proximity to parents in the face of these parental tendencies. In "the majority of cases," attentional/representational states are "likely preserved from infancy to adulthood (and transmitted from adult to infant) through this mechanism" (pp. 453–454). In this regard, Main (1995) suggested that for individuals classified in the two "organized" insecure categories (dismissing or preoccupied), "transference-like patterns of interaction between interviewer and interviewee resembling the respective interactions of dismissing–avoidant or preoccupied–resistant dyads are recapitulated within the [AAI]" (p. 443).

Coding and Classifying

Coding. Although the AAI itself was well-suited for the purposes of our study, Main's coding system was not. One disadvantage of that system was that it emphasizes the rules or strategies by which individuals gain or limit access to the contents of working models in the interview situation more so than the content itself. As is discussed in more detail in chapter 6, our findings in the ethnographic phase suggested the need to devise separate measures in the larger-sample phase of the content and quality-of-thought components of participants' AAIs. Another disadvantage of Main's coding system for our study was that it imposes a preexisting classification scheme on samples and does not allow for the discovery of new patterns.

Thus, in this study, we developed a two-pronged alternative to Main's scheme for coding the AAI. First, Anne L. Dean and assorted graduate students, independently wrote qualitative descriptions pertaining to both quality-of-thought and thematic content in the margins of interviews and then met as a group to reach consensus on these specific descriptors. From these specific descriptors, we developed higher order descriptors and ultimately "whole interview" quality-of-thought and content categories, properties of which are described in chapter 6.

The second prong of our coding system was a modification of a Q-sort coding procedure developed by Kobak (Kobak & Sceery, 1988; Kobak, Cole, Ferenz-Gillies, & Fleming, 1989; Kobak, Cole, Ferenz-Gillies, Fleming, & Gamble, 1993) for the AAI. Kobak's procedure entailed rating descriptive statements on a scale from 1 to 9 according to how well statements characterized a respondent's interview. However, whereas Kobak used a single deck of statements containing both content and quality-of-thought items to describe an interview, we separated content and quality-of-thought items into two decks. Quality-of-thought items retained in our deck consisted entirely of those from Kobak's deck; content items consisted of those from Kobak's deck plus some additional items written by our research group to reflect themes evident from our qualitative analyses that were not captured by any of Kobak's content items. Therefore, in our study, all forms of the AAI (teen, mother–mother, mother–teen) were sorted twice—once for quality of thought and once for content.[7]

Classifying. A first step in identifying patterns in respondents' Q-sort item scores was to subject them to principal components analyses. As described in Appendix A (Part B-1), three principal components analyses were performed for each interview type (mother–mother, mother–teen, teen). One analysis for each interview type was performed on quality-of-thought and content Q-sort item scores combined. The objective was to see whether the two item types would factor together or separate out into different factors. From these analyses, we determined that quality-of-thought and thematic content are indeed separable components of working models.[8]

---

[7] More details concerning the Q-sort procedure are described in Appendix A, section A.

[8] The rationale and results of these analyses are described in Appendix A, section B (1).

The second principal components analysis for each interview type was performed on quality-of-thought items alone, and the third was performed on content items alone. Scales derived from retained quality-of-thought (or content) factors were then analyzed according to internal consistency, and individuals' scores for scales meeting acceptable consistency criteria were then entered into cluster analyses to identify patterns.[9] For both quality-of-thought and content constructs, two or more cluster solutions were examined varying in the numbers of clusters requested. The numbers of clusters requested in these solutions approximated the numbers of categories identified through our qualitative analyses of interviews.

Classifications

Quality of thought. For the quality-of-thought construct, qualitative analyses revealed three categories closely matching descriptions of secure, preoccupied, and dismissing classifications in previous attachment studies, and a fourth category that we tentatively labeled *disorganized*. This category was similar to preoccupied in that respondents were excessively verbose, failed to maintain focus on a topic, were uncooperative in the interview, and generally were unable to reflect on or evaluate experiences insightfully. They differed from preoccupied respondents in reporting events with a decided lack of affect and in generating a more confused presentation overall, almost as an uninterrupted stream of consciousness. This mode was not restricted to topics concerning loss, abuse, or other traumas.

Attempts to arrive at a satisfactory level of intercoder reliability, however, were unsuccessful when the so-called disorganized category was included in the mix. Generally speaking, coders could not reliably differentiate the latter from the preoccupied category. When the disorganized category was dropped, high levels of intercoder agreement were reached on teen and mother–mother interviews (80% or better agreement for all pairs), but not for mother–teen interviews. Many of the mother–teen interviews fell into the "cannot classify" category described in Main (1995), in that mothers' quality of thought in describing their daughters' attachment relationships was inconsistent and depended on the topic they were addressing. Close examination of these interviews did not reveal a sufficiently clear pattern of inconsistency to draw firm conclusions. However, a subset of mothers who appeared secure in the bulk of the interview became preoccupied or disorganized when the topic of their daughters'

---

[9] More complete descriptions of methods used to determine internal consistency of scales, the compositions of retained scales, and patterns of centroids resulting from cluster analyses are found in Appendix A, section B (2-4).

adolescent sexuality was broached (either by themselves spontaneously or in response to interview questions added at the end).

Both three-group and four-group cluster analyses were requested for quality-of-thought Q-sorts for teen and mother–mother interviews. The three-group analyses yielded clusters with sufficient numbers of cases in each to allow for further analysis—clusters in which characteristics closely matched descriptions in the attachment literature and our qualitative analyses of secure, preoccupied, and dismissing patterns. The four-group analyses revealed clusters that were unevenly distributed and that were difficult to interpret in relation to our qualitatively derived categories or attachment research. As a consequence, we retained the three-cluster solutions.

Content. For the content construct, which we labeled *internal working models proper*, qualitative analyses revealed three main categories, each subdivided into two. These classifications were applicable and could be reliably differentiated (with 80% agreement or better) for teen and mother–mother interviews. They were labeled *deprived–acknowledged; deprived–denied; competitive–acknowledged; competitive–denied; mature, father–distant;* and *mature, father–close*. Descriptions of these are presented in chapter 6. Cluster analyses requesting from five to seven clusters identified patterns conforming descriptively to these categories for mother–mother interviews. For the teen cohort, the same classifications were derived, with the exception that only one competitive category emerged from cluster analyses.

For mother–teen content items, a four-group cluster analysis performed on content Q-sort factor scores yielded a variable labeled *mother representation*, consisting of three categories with sufficient numbers of cases: mother perceives daughter's relationship with herself as poor but better than with Dad (Bad Mom/Bad Dad), mother perceives daughter's relationship with Dad as better than the bad relationship daughter has with herself (Bad Mom/Good Dad), and mother perceives daughter's relationship with herself and with Dad as good (Good Mom/Good Dad).[10] The fourth group emerging from this analysis included two cases in which mother represented daughter's relationship with herself in glowing terms and with Dad in negative terms (Good Mom/Bad Dad). These cases were combined with those in the Bad Mom/Bad Dad group to yield a Mixed Mom/Bad Dad group.

---

[10] Our methods for coding and constructing categories from the AAI differed from both Main's and Kobak's (in that a different set of Q-items was used). Thus we cannot claim equivalence or comparability between our quality-of-thought construct and the attachment construct (quality of thought, state of mind, internal working model) developed in other studies. Findings emerging from this research, therefore, can be interpreted only in the context of our sample.

Validation of Quality-of-Thought and Content Classifications

Because mothers' and daughters' interviews were classified twice—once using qualitative methods and once using quantitative methods—and because these two sets of classifications were arrived at independently, the question of how well results from one method predict results from the other naturally arises. Separate discriminant function analyses of the mother–mother content, mother–mother quality of thought, teen content, teen quality of thought, and mother–teen content Q-sorts were conducted to answer this question. In each analysis, scores from the principal components analyses used to form clusters were entered as variables predicting to whole-interview, qualitatively derived classifications. As would be expected from the fact that we retained cluster solutions that most closely corresponded to categories resulting from qualitative analyses, hit rates from these analyses were exceedingly high (ranging between 86% and 99%). These numbers suggest a close parallel between the characteristics of interview classifications derived by multivariate analyses of Q-sort item scores and derived by qualitative analyses.

To further validate quality-of-thought classifications derived via Q-sorts and multivariate analyses, we classified respondents' interviews again by correlating their quality-of-thought Q-sort item scores with corresponding item scores from Kobak et al.'s (1989) secure–insecure and dismissing–preoccupied prototype sorts. Using Kobak et al.'s criteria, we grouped respondents into four categories: secure with dismissing tendencies, secure with preoccupied tendencies, insecure with dismissing tendencies, and insecure with preoccupied tendencies. The contingency table relating these four groupings to the three quality-of-thought groups derived from our cluster analyses is shown in Table 4-1.

The table shows that 86% of teens and 93% of moms classified by our cluster analyses as preoccupied were either classified as secure–preoccupied or insecure–preoccupied using Kobak's method. Ninety percent of teens and 91% of moms classified as dismissing by our cluster analyses were either secure–dismissing or insecure–dismissing according to Kobak's method. Ninety-two percent of teens and 85% of moms classified as secure by our cluster analyses were either secure–preoccupied or secure–dismissing according to Kobak et al.'s method. Cramer's V correlation coefficient summarizing the relations between these methods was .58, $p < .001$.

These findings suggest that our quality-of-thought construct bears some resemblance to the quality-of-thought component of internal working models described in other AAI studies, and thus lends support to Ward

Table 4-1 Comparison of Classifications Derived from Kobak's and the Cluster Methods

	Cluster Categories					
	Teens			Moms		
Kobak's Categories	Pre	Dis	Sec	Pre	Dis	Sec
Secure/Dismissing	0	5	3	2	1	5
Secure/Preoccupied	18	1	21	25	1	25
Insecure/Dismissing	4	23	1	0	19	4
Insecure/Preoccupied	7	3	1	3	1	1

Note. Pre = Preoccupied; Dis = Dismissing; Sec = Secure.

and Carlson's (1991) observation that "the characteristics of discourse and behavior that differentiate secure from insecure relationships appear to be robust across social class and maternal age" (p. 18).

Joint Mother–Daughter Interview

The joint mother–daughter interview was designed to assess the emotional content of mothers' and daughters' styles of communicating with one another. All dyads were asked to focus on relationship issues of their own choosing. The interviewer began by saying "You have both told us about your relationship with each other in the individual interviews. Now I'd like to ask you a few more questions while you are together. Could you tell me a little more about how you all get along? Either person can go first." Following this introductory remark, the primary role of the interviewer was to facilitate the flow of the discussion by reflecting back what had just been said in the form of a question or asking general questions such as "How has your relationship changed over the years?" or "Are there any areas that cause conflict?" For dyads in which daughters had become pregnant, the interviewer directed the dyad if necessary to the topic of the pregnancy and the baby, asking about feelings, caretaking arrangements, changes in the mother–daughter relationship as a result of the pregnancy, and hopes for the future. For the most part, however, partners in the dyad chose who spoke when, how much, and about what, and interviewer questions and prompts were kept to a minimum.[11]

---

[11] Joint interviews were coded using the *Analysis of Family Interview* (Nathanson, Baird, & Jemail, 1986) described in detail in Appendix B, section B (1-a).

5

Family Environments and Cultural Schemas in the Larger Sample

FAMILY ENVIRONMENTS

Our ethnographic data suggested that pregnancies among poor, unwed African American teenagers are not uniform phenomena, as is often assumed in discussions of this topic. Rather, they occur in multiple, intersecting contexts within which superficially similar behavior patterns take on differing underlying meanings.

In this chapter, the first focus is on family-of-origin environmental contexts for adolescent pregnancy. Those theoreticians (e.g., LeVine, 1982) who hold to the "separate but intersecting" view of relations between cultural and psyche might argue that family environments, more so than any other constructs measured empirically in the larger-sample phase, lend themselves to conceptualization as separate from or "external" to the individual psyche. As external contexts, mothers' and daughters' family-of-origin environments might be conceptualized as nested outer layers in the adolescent pregnancy system within which mental representational and behavioral phenomena are embedded. Further, as external entities, family environments might be thought of as describable in so-called objective terms that would be agreed on by most competent observers. In support of this view, family environment classifications as we operationally defined them in the larger-sample phase incorporated some features that are independently verifiable by individuals other than the interviewee. These were "structural" features such as numbers of parents heading the household at the time of the interview, parents' marital and employment histories, and numbers of times mothers or daughters left their family households to live elsewhere (a measure of family stability).

Table 5-1 Cluster Centroids for Mother and Teen Family Environment Variables

Classification	Mother			Teen		
	Nuclear F	Ex-Kin	n	Nuclear F	Ex-Kin	n
Downward - 1	-1.67	-1.45	6	-.92	-2.12	6
Downward - 2	-1.32	.54	18	-.92	.09	33
Traditional	.65	.72	34	.48	1.21	17
Upward	.41	-.91	28	.96	-.43	31

Note. Nuclear F = Nuclear family variable; Ex-Kin = Extended Kin Network variable.

Components of the family environment construct having to do with networking characteristics of extended families, however, do not lend themselves as easily to characterizations as objective or external. These components include mothers' and daughters' memories of incidents in which extended kin provided services or support, material or otherwise; assessments of the composition and extensiveness of the kin network; and assessments of the degree to which kin networks are felt as truly viable and supportive. These memories, judgments, and feelings are influenced as much by internal as external factors. Thus, rather than representing a separate, external context surrounding separate, internal contexts, the family environment construct as we have constituted here is better thought of as representing one pole of an internal–external dialectical relation.

The primary questions asked in regard to family-of-origin environments in this chapter are, do the same constellations of characteristics discovered in the ethnographic phase (downwardly mobile, traditional, and upwardly mobile) adequately characterize the descriptions of mothers and daughters in the larger sample, are modifications of these earlier descriptions necessary, and are entirely different descriptions needed?

Our findings indicated that, with some modifications and elaborations, patterns in structural and extended-kin measures identified through cluster analyses for both mother and daughter cohorts matched descriptions of downwardly mobile, traditional, and upwardly mobile families presented in chapters 2 and 3. Four-group cluster analyses using SPSS-X Quick Cluster Program (SPSS, Inc., 1988) were performed on mothers' and teens' standardized scores for the nuclear family and extended-kin variables. These analyses yielded the patterns of cluster centroids shown in Table 5-1.

The first two clusters in the table have negative loadings on the nuclear family variable, a defining characteristic of the downwardly mobile family described in chapter 3. In one variant of this downwardly mobile family type (downward - 1), respondents described a limited extended-kin network, whereas in the second (downward—2), respondents described at least a moderately extensive network. Because of the small numbers of both teens and mothers in the first variant, we combined it with the second in subsequent analyses. The third cluster in Table 1 has positive loadings on both nuclear and extended-kin variables—both characteristics of the traditional family type described in chapter 3. The fourth pattern has a positive loading on the nuclear but a negative loading on the extended-kin variable, characteristics of the upwardly mobile family type described in chapter 3. Thus, cluster analyses performed on individuals' scores for the two composite variables revealed patterns corresponding to the three family environment types.[1]

As seen in Table C-2 (Appendix C, section B), downwardly mobile families in both cohorts were distinguished by the absence of two parents in the home, the rarity of stable marriages that occurred before first pregnancies, unstable residential patterns, and heavy reliance on governmental financial assistance. Within the downwardly mobile category, however, families were a heterogeneous group. Whereas many were headed by a single mother alone, others included single mothers and their own mothers and/or grandmothers, sisters, or boyfriends who may or may not have been fathers of the mothers' children. Families described in Burton's (1990, 1993) ethnographic study of the Gospel Hill community (i.e., households composed of multigenerations of women without stable male partners) are included in this group.

Traditional families in both mother and daughter cohorts combined two-parent households with a kin network experienced as both extensive and supportive. Traditional family households were also a heterogeneous group, some headed by mother and father alone and others including members of either parent's extended family. Some traditional families in this study, for example, included multigenerations of women (the teen, her mother, and her mother's mother or the teen, her children, and her mother) in combination with a stable male (mother's or grandmother's husband), thus constituting a variant of the multigenerational family category not described in Burton's (1990, 1993) research.

Upwardly mobile families in both cohorts combined two-parent households with extended-kin networks experienced as less extensive and less supportive than traditional extended-kin networks and less functional than networks of downwardly mobile and traditional families in the sense

---

[1] Table C-1 in Appendix C, section A, shows percentages of older and younger mothers and teens classified as downwardly mobile, traditional, or upwardly mobile. Table C-2, Appendix C, section B, shows patterns of mothers' and teens' responses on items included in composite variables as a function of family environment classifications.

of providing alternative places of residence for children or teens. Upwardly mobile households in both cohorts, however, were as likely as both of these other family types to include other "kin."

Traditional families in the mother cohort, however, differed qualitatively from those in the teen cohort. The teen variant of the traditional family more closely resembled the downwardly mobile than upwardly mobile family type, whereas the mother variant of the traditional family more closely resembled the upwardly mobile than downwardly mobile family type. Teen traditional families were less likely than mother traditional families to be headed by parents employed full time and who were married prior to the birth of the first child, less likely to be headed by two parents, and more likely to have involved separations of respondents from birth parents. Moreover, as seen in Table C-1 (Appendix C-A), more teen families were categorized as downwardly mobile than younger mother families, who in turn were categorized more often as downwardly mobile than older mother families. Although downwardly mobile mothers were most likely to have downwardly mobile daughters (58%), and upwardly mobile mothers were most likely to have upwardly mobile daughters (46%), traditional mothers were more likely to have downwardly mobile daughters (47%) than either traditional (24%) or upwardly mobile (29%) daughters.

Significant numbers of traditional African American families in this rural area of the South, therefore, have gradually but perceptibly merged into the downwardly mobile form. On the other hand, the failure of our data to demonstrate comparable transformations of traditional into upwardly mobile family forms may be more a reflection of the restriction of the sample to poor families than of the absence of this trend. In a manner of speaking, families that have become upwardly mobile since the era in which the older mother cohort was born may have priced themselves out of our market.

These findings are consistent with McAdoo's (1988b) suggestion that extended-kin networks support poor African Americans' efforts to attain the educational and occupational skills needed for movement into the middle class. Viable extended-kin networks (the traditional family) were associated with households headed by stable married couples, suggesting a reciprocal relation between these two characteristics. Extended-kin networks are strengthened by the presence of two adults within individual households, and the presence of two adults within individual households is supported by the resources available within the extended-kin network. We suggest that for poor African American families like those in our sample, inexorable trends toward deterioration of extended-kin networks and replacement of two-parent households with one-parent households will make the transition to the middle class more problematic.

CULTURALLY CONSTITUTED SCHEMAS OF ADOLESCENT SEXUALITY

A proposition much discussed within cognitive anthropology is that individuals form cognitive and emotional schemas based on their shared experiences in a cultural environment (D'Andrade & Strauss, 1992; Schwartz, White, & Lutz, 1993). Culturally constituted cognitive schemas, as defined by cognitive anthropologists, are complex, hierarchically organized entities representing thoughts, feelings, and actions relevant to the past, present, and future. Embedded in these complexes are desires and goals, both conscious and unconscious. Schemas thus are both motivational and descriptive (Strauss, 1992).

Using this cognitive anthropological perspective as a theoretical framework, I hypothesized that mothers of poor African American adolescent daughters, who themselves may have grown up in downwardly mobile or traditional family environments and who themselves perhaps were adolescent mothers, construct implicit cognitive schemas incorporating adolescent pregnancies as a subordinate goal in the service of the superordinate goal of forming and maintaining networks. Such schemas may be manifested through mothers' verbal, behavioral, and emotional responses to daughters' incipient and actual adolescent sexuality, which responses may serve as communications to daughters regarding the desirability of unwed adolescent pregnancies. From this perspective, mothers' schemas and implicit communications would constitute connecting links between what the group (members of a given family environment niche) implicitly knows is useful for economic survival and what individual girls come to feel and understand as desirable.

Preliminary evidence in favor of this hypothesis was obtained in the ethnographic phase. Virtually all mothers we talked to in the ethnographic phase, regardless of family environment context, verbalized the belief that adolescent pregnancy is unwanted and detrimental to the quest for desired middle-class status. Many also denounced pregnancies of unwed women as immoral. The actions and emotional responses of some mothers, however, paradoxically and simultaneously communicated the opposite belief that adolescent pregnancies are desirable. This message was communicated through inconsistencies among mothers' words, emotional displays, and deeds. A standard script, differing from telling to telling only in minor details, illustrated these inconsistences. The script generally read like this:

Mother reacts with excitement, great concern, and increased attentiveness to daughter at the news of daughter's menstruation.

Mother closely monitors daughter's monthly periods and communicates the belief that daughter is "doing something," a belief contradicted by daughter's assertion that she is "doin' nothing." Mother may take daughter for frequent check-ups at the health clinic to determine her pregnancy state. Mother states rules regarding daughter's activities with boys, but often lapses in her monitoring of these activities, as daughter spends time alone with her "boyfriend" at his mother's, an older sister's, or other relatives' houses. Mother may give daughter either a lot or very little information about sex, pregnancy or birth control, but explicitly tells daughter that birth control pills can mess up her insides, as they did to mother's insides. When daughter "inexplicably" becomes pregnant, mother is distraught and angry, and daughter cowers in fear. Through her anger and shame, however, mother concedes that "what's done is done," and admonishes daughter to face up to her coming responsibilities. As the time for the baby's birth draws near, mother relents and both she and daughter anticipate the event with joy. After the baby is born, mother and daughter state that the pregnancy was unwanted, but now that the baby is here, "there's nothing to do but love it."

In this script, the explicit message "Don't get pregnant" competes with the implicit message "Pregnancy is expected and desired." The standardization of this script in this poor, African American community points to its shared cultural origins.

In the larger sample of mothers and daughters interviewed in the second phase of the research, analyses[2] revealed two general categories of cultural schemas reflecting inconsistencies or consistencies among mothers' professed attitudes about daughters' adolescent sexuality; their giving of information about sex, pregnancy, and birth control; and their emotional attitudes toward daughters in the joint-interview session. Both kinds of schemas—inconsistent and consistent—could be subdivided into two.

In the first subcategory of inconsistent schema, hereby labeled the

---

[2] To search for patterns in mothers' and daughters' attitudes and beliefs about matters relating to daughters' sexuality and in their emotional responses to each other when conversing about such matters, we first used principal components factor analyses to construct composite variables from dyads' scores on sex and pregnancy items and joint-interview scales. Scores from two principal components labeled *mother gives information* and *mother is strict* were derived from analyses of sex and pregnancy items, and scores from two principal components labeled *mother engagement* and *conflict* were derived from analyses of Analysis of Family Interview items. Dyads' scores on the four variables were entered into a four-group cluster analysis, and patterns of cluster centroids representing four cultural schemas emerged. Details of these analyses are presented in Appendix B, section B.

restrictive but noninformative schema, mothers portray themselves as vocal in describing the dangers of boys and in the setting of rules restricting daughters' activities with boys. At the same time, mothers communicate ambivalence about setting rules; convey a sense of helplessness to interviewers and to daughters about their capacity to enforce rules; omit telling daughters essential information about sex, pregnancy, and birth control; and maintain an emotionally disengaged attitude when discussing problematic issues with daughter. Numerous rationalizations are offered for why rules cannot be enforced and why information cannot be given.

In the second subcategory of inconsistent schema, labeled *informative but nonrestrictive*, mothers convey detailed specific information to daughters about sex, pregnancy, and birth control but are lax in establishing and enforcing rules regulating daughters' activities with boys. Mothers in these dyads adopt an accusatory attitude toward daughters in the joint-interview session while maintaining an emotionally disengaged attitude.

In the first subcategory of consistent schema, hereby labeled the *restrictive and informative* schema, mothers profess the need to establish and enforce rules; convey specific detailed information about sex, pregnancy, and contraceptives; are confrontational with daughters with regard to their activities; and maintain an engaged emotional attitude reflecting an attempt to control daughters' behavior. In the second subcategory, labeled the *nonrestrictive and noninformative* schema, mothers are emotionally engaged with daughters while adopting a nonrestrictive, relatively uninformative, and nonaccusatory stance with regard to daughters' adolescent sexuality.

Some properties of cultural schemas, however, cannot be conveyed by numbers. What gets lost in the translation of narratives to numbers are the many, usually subtle ways in which mothers simultaneously communicate two different messages to daughters and to interviewers, the ways in which daughters simultaneously process and understand both sets of incoming messages, and the many ways in which these contradictions are reconciled in the minds of those who are thinking and feeling them. These particular qualitative properties of mothers' and daughters' minds defy translation into numbers. In the following section excerpts are presented from one mother–never-pregnant daughter dyad for each of the four schemas; thereafter, the properties of schemas overall as derived from qualitative analyses of interviews are summarized.

Inconsistent: Restrictive but Noninformative

The mother of a 15-year-old never-pregnant girl is vague with regard to the information she gave her daughters about sex, pregnancy, and birth control when they first got their periods: "I told 'em if they do it, don't go out there and get pregnant. . . . I just tell 'em to keep their dress down. And that if they go mess around on their private parts they'll get pregnant." This impression of vagueness is confirmed by her 15-year-old daughter, who states that mother did not tell her much of anything.

Mother's attitudes about rules are fraught with ambivalence and contradiction. Mother and daughter are both clear that mother has not given daughter permission to date and will not until daughter becomes 16, even though both acknowledge that daughter has had boyfriends. Although mother denies daughter permission to date, mother is not sure that stringent rules are warranted, because "you can't keep kids tied down to the house all the time." Daughter, meanwhile, is aware of both mother's prohibitions and the fact that they are not firm because boys can (and do) come by the house. Mother feels that despite her rules, daughter is out of control and that she is powerless to do anything about it; sometimes mother believes she is not doing a very good job with daughter:

> She doesn't have permission (to date), but I think she has been sneaking out. 'Cause she got sick one time. Thought maybe she might have got something from somebody. That's what I thought but I didn't know for sure cause I wasn't in there when the doctor examined her. He said she had an infection. He didn't say what kind that she had. Yeah, and he gave her some antibiotics. I asked her, she said she hadn't been with anybody. I told her the only way you can get it is you been messing with someone. That's when she got down sick, when she was going out with friends. She'll be gone a whole day, and come back at 10:00. . . . She doesn't admit to anything. You ask her, she'll say she hasn't.

Daughter, in the meantime, proves the validity of mother's belief that "you can't keep kids tied down to the house all the time" by arranging to have sex with her boyfriend in his mother's house.

Mother justifies not telling daughter about birth control because she is not yet old enough to date, even though she strongly suspects that daughter is currently "doin' something." Mother anticipates telling daughter about birth control pills when she is old enough to date, but at the same time remembers her own bad experience with them:

> They [her daughters] have all kind of stuff for birth control. They know about those. Mostly from me because uh, when I was having kids, I tried birth control pills. But they didn't work for me. They made me gain weight, and everything else, so I had to get off of 'em.

Daughter indicates that she has received mother's message that birth control pills are undesirable, and states that she would not use them: "(I don't know) that much, but you know, that it prevent pregnancy. I wouldn't use birth control. I guess he'd have to use the condom or something."

Mother's primary mode of reconciling what she explicitly states should not be happening with what she implicitly knows is happening is to claim ignorance of much of what is going on in daughter's life. Mother is unsure about many things, such as whether daughter is sneaking out and messing around, what grades daughter is making in school, whether daughter has been pregnant, or whether daughter has a specific boyfriend. If things happen, they happen when mother is asleep, and therefore she does not know about them:

> To tell you the truth, I don't know (when [she] might "talk" to boys). When I'm tired from doing all the housework, I'm going to sleep. . . . Uh, I'm not sure about that because we got a rule that nobody goes anywhere while we're sleeping. Like if I do housework, I rarely get help from some of 'em, some of the time. And I do most of the housework, and I get tired. [Has she been pregnant?] I don't think she has. . . . She talks to boys on the phone, but I don't know um, if she has any specific boy that she's interested in to go out with when she gets 16. . . . Oh, one boy [boyfriend's name] she keep mentioning. I think he's 20. Maybe 22. . . . Well, he had came in the house one time when I was sleeping, late at night, the one they call [boyfriend's name]. And she went out there. I didn't know none of that had happened 'cause I was sleeping. He didn't came in, he stayed outside, and she went outside to talk to him. And my husband went out there and told him she's not getting no company that late at night. And besides, she's not old enough to have no boyfriend now. (She) got mad as usual. Went up to her room as usual.

In this way, mother expounds one set of standards when she is awake but tacitly agrees to another when she is asleep.

Inconsistent: Informative but Nonrestrictive

In this dyad, the usual tables are turned with respect to mother's and daughter's interest in daughter's adolescent sexuality. Mother is more invested than daughter in the prospects of daughter's potential adolescent pregnancy. Mother gives explicit information to daughter about sex and pregnancy:

After I found out, you know, she was having her period, I talked,
I sat down and talked to her. I said "I have a book. This is what
men and women do. This is what they call sex. They have a relation . . . man inserts his penis in her vagina." She looked at me
all funny and everything. [laugh] I said "Whenever he ejaculate
in her, the sperm will travel up. If it meets the egg, she becomes
pregnant."

Mother, however, remains uninvolved in the setting of rules, implying that
because daughter has expressed no interest in having sex, rules and birth
control are unnecessary: "And she said 'Well, I don't wanna become pregnant, me. I ain't never gonna do that.' [laughs] I never had no problem
with her since, you know."

At the same time, however, mother adopts an accusatory attitude
toward daughter in the joint-interview session, implying that daughter is
"doing something." Mother states that she would put daughter on birth
control if necessary, but that she is scared of the pills:

I was scared they [her daughters] was gonna react like I had. Even
they was takin 'em, they was gonna get pregnant. Or either, well,
I had to get my stomach pumped one time from birth control
pills, because they give infection in the stomach.

Mother seems disappointed that daughter does not have a boyfriend and
communicates irritation about daughter's own worry about the dangers
of walking past bars late at night:

That's what I'm saying, she never really went out with any boys.
Like they would like have a hop or something, she'd be at the
hop, you know. Like the boys would be there, and she'd be there
with them. But you know, like uh, he came by one night, this guy
[boyfriend's name] came by one Christmas, before Christmas he
came by. So she introduced me to him and everything. And she
would talk to him on the phone or something. I said "[Daughter's
name] have a boyfriend at last!" But she said "Mama, I don't like
that boy. He's not coming here no more." So he never came
back. . . . Uh . . . the hop is usually over for 1:00, and they be
home. . . . She comes straight home. I don't have no problem with
her hanging out and everything. She comes straight home. And
if she goes to, like I said, my cousin owns a bar, if she goes to, she
don't really go to the bar, they have a bar with a house onto it . . .
but they have another house they stay in, she'll be in there, and
she'll call me "Mama, come meet me cause I'm coming home and

I don't wanna pass by the bar by myself." So I have to get the other kids out the bed and walk over to bring her home. Oh, OK . . . say about 12:00.

Mother lets daughter know that she, mother, would be unable to prevent daughter from having sex if she wanted it and that if daughter just happened to become pregnant, mother would encourage daughter to go ahead and have the baby:

I figure, you know, if she want to have sex, I can't stop it. I'm not with her 24 hours a day. . . . You know, she tell me "Mama," she used to tell me "what's an abortion?" "Ma, if I would get pregnant, would you give me an abortion?" I said "Do what? Abortion?" I said "I didn't do it with you. I had you. My Mama had seven children. And she had all seven of those. If I had to have seven I would have 'em. Cause if the Lord didn't want you to have it, it wouldn't stay here." So she said "You mean that?" I said "Yes, I mean it." She said "I wouldn't do that anyway." She was just trying me. [laughs] She does that a lot.

Daughter, in the meantime, acknowledges mother's willingness to give information about sex, pregnancy, and birth control and is aware of mother's concern that when a girl becomes 17, the dangers of pregnancy are particularly pressing.

A lot of times I asked her questions, basic questions, and she'd tell me. Um, in the beginning, it was stupid questions like "Well, Mama, why you got pregnant? How you got pregnant? When? Where?" But um, after I saw she wasn't answering those, I started asking decent questions like um, if I hear something at school, I'd hear somebody say um, if you have sex a day before your period come day, you automatically pregnant. And I would ask her, and she would explain it. And um, let's see, another question, um, "Can you get pregnant before you even see your period, just by a boy you having sex with a person? Can you um, get pregnant by not even, like him not even entering you? Just messing around?" Um. And about birth control a lot. I asked her, um, I've always asked questions, but um, there was once a conversation between her and my aunt, and they said, um, that since I was 17, they thought it was time that she should talk to me about it. So, um, she was telling me. She didn't just tell me about the pills. She was telling me about um, sponge, and contraceptive gels, or whatever you insert in you. And um, the diaphragm. And [mumbling].

But um, she asked me if I thought I should be on 'em, and I told her no, because I, you know, I wasn't worried about, I'm not into sex, so I'm not really into birth control. And, um, that was that.

Juxtaposed with this acknowledgment of mother's interest and concern about the dangers of boys and sex, however, is daughter's awareness that mother has imposed few restrictions on her dating:

[Permission to date?] Yeah! [Boyfriend?] Yeah, but I never took it as serious. Just a little case of puppy love. I could never say I felt serious enough about a boy to say um . . . everybody's just into having sex. I never felt serious enough to have sex with a boy. (Stay out) 'til about 1:30. But um, really, I don't have a curfew at all.

And despite mother's anticipation that daughter might just happen to have sex and become pregnant, daughter is of the opinion that things do not just happen:

[Future for self?] Um, a very independent one. One where I plan to get married and have a family, but um, I do want to have a career of my own. And um, I don't wanna be in a marriage where the husband is very dominant. I wanna be involved in some choices. And um, in most of the choices, you know. (Want my children) to be aware of the things around them. Not naive, trusting in anybody or any situation. To um, be aggressive. And go after what they want. Don't sit around and let things happen for you. You have to make things happen.

Consistent: Restrictive and Informative Schemas

The mother of this never-pregnant daughter portrays herself as adamant with respect to protecting daughter from single-minded boys and as willing to go to almost any lengths to accomplish this task:

If she wants to go somewhere, sometimes I be skeptical. It's nowhere, not a date, or not out-of-town, you know, sometimes it's "Can we go to Pizza Hut after the game, or can we go to McDonald's, or can I go to a dance?" Now I've been very skeptical about things like that, like a dance. I'll let her go with her friends to Pizza Hut and I feel at ease about that. I'll say, what time am I coming to get you, or call me when you are ready. So, I mean like I said, she's 17, but in a public place, it's not too much you can do, you know. Of course there are boys around, because they will always be stuck together. But as far as school functions, such as dances, now one particular instance she asked me to go, and I didn't let her. I didn't let her go. And she ended up going to McDonald's, with you know, two or three other friends. Well that was fine, I'm glad I didn't let her go to that dance, because there are too many outside older people, and before that night was over, they ended up fighting in the streets. I followed my right mind on that one. So, that was just out. No, no, no outside dances, if it something at school, fine. Well she, you know, she has been to the Spring dance and what have you. After school, that's fine. Uh, outside, No. (Okay, um).

An anecdote clearly illustrates this mother's determination:

Now last year she got involved with an older guy, but he was living with his grandmother, like two houses or so from my mother. And he had come from New Orleans, he knew all the ropes, she was a minor. Now I would see her talk to him, you know, across the fence, but never had I given my approval for anything more. She just assumed that I thought it was okay. She was 16. Just, just last, just last year, year before last, 15 or 16. So, she continued to talk to him, so I, I told her I didn't want her to talk to him. And she disobeyed me. She was still talking to him but had me thinking he was somebody else. So, one day, she came home from school, and at this time my sister saw it, she was with my mother, they came, they went to the same school and got home together. So I called for her, he said she wasn't there. This is strange. Now that really upset me because it was nothing I could do until my husband came home, like an hour and a half later. So when he did, when he did come, and we headed toward my mother's house, I saw her standing outside, talking to him. Well really, she was sitting in the car, talking to him. So I said, keep your head straight, you know, because you know, the more you rebel, the more they rebel against you. So, I ended up, I really ended up putting her on birth control. And I ended up going to the police for him, because he was very disrespectful and ignored me. I say well, if I can't stop you, I know who can. And that, that's stopped him. That definitely stopped him. And by my talking to her, stopped her, brought her to her senses. Because I told her like it was. I mean, he was 20 something years old. He was going to college. I said, "Do you actually believe he is going to all these young college women and his mind is dead set on you?" I say "You better wake up and smell the flowers." Now this was like in February, of last year. December, he got married. I say, "You want to tell me he loved you?" So, that, that kind of brought, I had to do some talking, and she was in a state of depression, so I guess he really blew her mind. But I had to do some talking to bring her back to her senses, because she actually thought he loved her. And that was like a first time, she had talked to boys before, but that was really a first time experience for her. So, she okay now. And it didn't take her long, because I wasn't gonna let it take her long to get over that. And I, I, I meant that. I mean, she's my daughter, I have to look out for her welfare until, until she becomes of age to take care of herself. . . . She's my responsibility. And he was just so dead set, he thought that he had her where he wanted her. I couldn't control her feelings. I couldn't help the way she felt. I couldn't change the way she felt. I say, we'll see about that! So, I see him every now and then now, because his grandparents still live next to my mother. But if I ever have to go to the police again, I'm going, I'm going. And I don't care who doesn't like it, because . . . well there's one house in-between their house and my mother's. And there are young men that live over there. But ever since they moved there and found my mother there, they have been respectable young men. And he told them, that I'm trigger happy . . . All I want him to do is open his mouth and say one word to my daughter, and that's what I meant. That's what I meant. And I still mean it. I'll go to bat for her.

Mother's actions of giving daughter specific information about sex, pregnancy, and birth control and of putting daughter on birth control are consistent with this attitude:

(I put her on birth control pills). I told her that it was not OK for her to go out and have sex (just because she was on the pill), but that it was a protection, because she was not going to be around me all of her life. And I wanted her to use her head. I say, this does not mean that you can go out and have all the fun you want. This is just a precaution, because, I think she had sex with him. I'm not sure. She told me she did, and she told me that he used a condom. But I told her a condom didn't mean nothing to me and I told her it was by the grace of God that she didn't get pregnant. She was lucky, because it take but a split second. I just laid it on the line. I say that was all he was after, because you are young and that's all he wants. I couldn't, she couldn't, I couldn't get through. She just claimed that he cared for her so much. "But he love me momma, I know it." I say girl, "You're crazy!" [laughs] I just, I'm just telling you, that's because (you tell me, you tell me) that's the way I talk. I say, "Are you out of your mind?" I say, "All of these young women they have up on Southern campus, and you're telling me he loves you?" I, I really told her good. She wasn't despondent, you know, but you could tell she was down and everything. But I told her things, and that's what I intended to so. So I mean, since then, she has, she has alot of guys, you know, classmates she talks to on the phone. She has a boyfriend now, and he has been to see her. She's never been to his house, but she won't get there unless his mother is home! [laughs] She won't. And I mean that. Because he asked her, was he, was she gonna come and see him before she went on the trip. I told her to tell him, whenever his momma phones, she can go. As long as his mother is home. And as long as I know she is going to be there.

Although mother does not remember much about what she first told daughter about sex, pregnancy, and birth control, daughter does:

(Mother told daughter at age 13 that) it [sex] wasn't really a nice thing to do, and that I would be ready for it when, when I thought I was. And, um, that it was my decision, but my decision is when I'm ready. [How did you get information about sex?] By, um, checking books out from the library and reading them all. She helped me with it. She would help me look for the books. And we'd sit down and, after I read them, we'd sit down and talk about them.

Daughter understands and complies with mother's prescriptions concerning birth control:

She [mother] said that it was, it wasn't an invitation to go out and have sex. It was a precaution. . . . She basically told me about the birth control pill. Well, I have some birth control pills. (Got them) to the Health Unit. They're about ninety percent effective. Well, you take them the same time every day, you take them in the morning.

Consistent: Nonrestrictive and Noninformative

Mother's emotional attitude of nonadversarial engagement with daughter in the joint-interview session is combined with a nonrestrictive, relaxed, and accepting attitude about daughter's entrance into puberty and dating. Mother provides rudimentary information about sex, pregnancy, and contraception in a context of trust that daughter will use her best judgment in deciding about these matters. Mother's attitude is that daughter need not be strictly monitored or controlled. Also implied is mother's expectation that daughter will want to model herself after mother and that daughter shares mother's values:

> (I told her) "Well, some boys be honest with you. Some don't. Well, if anybody ask you for sex, you have a mouth to say 'no.' Because you're too young for that. Try to wait until you're married. Or, you know, at least until you're married." And I told her what I did. I was . . . I told her I was 19 when I got pregnant with her. I was still a virgin then. I hadn't never been . . . I had boyfriends, yeah, but her Daddy was the first. And when I did, I was pregnant, I got pregnant. I told her all of that. I told her how some boys do, all they want is your body, and fool you, and tell you they love you and all that. And then once they get what they want, they don't have nothing to do with you. She understood all that. And I told her, I said "Well, I can't tell you what to do, but I pray to God you listen at me. You don't go give your body away. Try to wait until you be your own woman. Get married and then, because . . ." I told her, I say "You don't have to follow in my steps, but I hope you do. I was 19. I got pregnant with you. I was a virgin when I slept with your Daddy. Then we married. I want you to . . ." I told her I went with a boy for two years and a half, and he, he living around here now. He couldn't tell nobody if I'm a man or a woman. And we went together 2 years. Two years and a half. And some people say "Oh, girl, you . . ." I said "Well, I could put my hand on the Bible and tell you that's true. So can he." I told her all that.
> [Permission to date?] Oh, yeah, but she don't. [laughs] She don't go anywhere. [Curfew?] Well, at least to 12, 12:30. That's what I used to tell her at that time, but she never did go like, like I said, they used to go riding. And I remember her saying they went to a show. They'll go ride out, and they'll come back home. We'll get our cold drink, our potato chips, we sit there, we play us a little game of some kind of Spades, this game they call the Spades. We'll play Spades together, me, her, her boyfriend, my other

daughter. We get there, we just like a family. That's all we do. She don't go to hops and, I never had a problem with her with hops. Like they have the school hops. She never did fool with that. I think [daughter's name] might have went about once or twice. I'm not sure, but I'd say about once or twice.

And birth control pills, I never was for that. I just don't. I took birth control pills, and when I was taking 'em, they messed my period up. I wouldn't see it some time for 2 and 3 months, then sometimes I didn't see my period for a whole year. So I told her like this, I said "If you decide, I hope you trust the Lord. You'll be on your own. But I'm not gonna put you on pills." I never did put my kids on pills. And I'm not planning on putting 'em on no pills. She's 19 now, like I told her, I hope and trust the Lord she gonna make something out of her life. I don't want her to get pregnant, but if that's what happens, well, she her own woman now. She can support herself. But I still preach that I'd rather for her to go make a career or something. Do something with her life. Don't just pop up with babies. Ummum.

But once she told me the boy that she go with now, and before she finished school, she told me, she came to me, she said "Mama, I don't know if you gonna believe me. I know you ain't gonna believe me. I'm a virgin. I ain't never had sex. He told me he loved me. He told me like this here. But he can wait." "Is that what he told you?" She said "Yeah. And that's what I told him. If he love me, he can wait. I waited for him when he went and made something out of his life, and he can wait for me." So he told her he wasn't gonna push her, and he wasn't gonna force her. I haven't talked to her lately about it, but before she, about a week before she graduated, she told me she still a virgin. That's when she went to this club for virgin people. She said she still a virgin. She told me "Mama, you don't have to worry about nothing. I ain't crazy."

[Club?] Uh, this garden club. It's for the virgins . . . if you're a virgin . . . this kind of club . . . Uhuh, they have it right, right here. Yeah, it was here, and she went to that. Well, all I know, they was telling me it was for girls who were still virgins. And, they have white dresses and all, white gowns . . . and things like that. Uhuh, yeah, that's what she told me, she's still a virgin, so. And deep down in my heart, I really believe she is. I don't have no doubt about that. If she isn't, she be done fooled her mama. 'Cause I do not have doubts about her.

[If she did become sexually active?] I don't know. She might tell me. She'd have to go to a clinic. She'll be able to get (birth control

pills) on her own. Uhuh. Yeah, she'll be 19 in March, so she
wouldn't need my permission. But I don't think she'll go to birth
control pills. I really don't think so. [Wish for her?] To stay just
like she is. [laughs] I wouldn't want nothing else to change. . . . I
wouldn't want her to change in no way. I'd wish that she could
be happy. Find if this is the right boy for her. And have her a nice
career where she can. . . . If something go wrong with them, she'll
have something to fall back on. Like I always did tell 'em, I want
'em to be like their certain way. But like I'm on welfare, and I
don't want them to have to do that. I want them to get an education so if something go down between husband and wife, whatever, they have something to get by on. They don't fall on welfare
and depend on that. That's all I pray to God for. Being nice, 'cause
I'm nice. And being herself. That's all. She's like me in a lot of
ways, certain ways. Like she have some part of me, and some part
of her Daddy. So . . .

Daughter recognizes mother's beliefs that pregnancy is not one of the
"good" things that can happen to an adolescent girl and that daughter
can be trusted to make her own decisions. Daughter remembers that
mother did not tell her much about sex or pregnancy because mother did
not think daughter was interested. Daughter takes pride in making responsible decisions and looks forward to a time when she is old enough to have
those things that she wants from life:

I know I get more money now (that I'm older) [laughs], than I
used to get. And I see boys. [Curfew?] Well, it's just like be back
at a respectable time. It's not like you can't go, or you don't need
to go . . . or some other time. It's just be back at a respectable
time. . . . Well, when I started dating, I still wouldn't go anywhere.
I didn't like going places. But if I would go, it wouldn't be
nowhere else unless we'd go to the movies. And most of the time
I would go out, I would go with someone older than me. And
someone that's responsible for their self so they can be responsible for me. I'd come home like 10, 10:30.
I was 13 when I first started my menstruation. . . . She [Mother]
just started telling me how to handle myself, and what to do,
what not to do. And what a young girl would want to know, or
would have to know, told me all about that. I was scared. I did-
n't know what was going on. Well, she was saying getting pregnant wasn't one of the good things, for sure. It wasn't one of the
good things, getting pregnant. [What did Mom tell you about
how a girl gets pregnant?] Really, she said things, but she didn't

come straight out and say how a girl gets pregnant. She'll say like messing with a guy. One of my friends, she was pregnant at the time. She didn't know what she was doing. And she asked me, and I went and asked my Mama sister cause I didn't know what to tell her [Mother]. So I asked my Mama sister, and she had had a child already, so I knew she had to know something. So she told us about the egg and the sperm, and what causes it. . . . I guess (Mother) didn't tell me 'cause I didn't go nowhere. I just stayed home. I guess she felt she didn't have to tell me.

[And did you find out about these things anywhere else?] Yeah, I did a research paper on teenage pregnancy. And I found most of the things in the library. And from my English teacher. I think um, a girl gets pregnant by having a boy enter her, I don't know how you say it. Just lets his sperm enter her, she becomes pregnant. And she's not on no birth control, or . . . whatever.

[Mother tell about birth control?] She said it's not good. She didn't use it . . . she doesn't like it. And um, she wouldn't want her children to be on birth control until like 18 or 19. She said when she got 'em, she was um, I think 18, and she got right off 'em . . . cause they would make her sick. And she said birth control is not good for all people. They blow some people up. And um, like that, and make some sick. They made her sick.

[Boyfriend?] We're gonna get married when I make about 24. And I would like to have a little girl, a nice house, and a good bit of money.

PROPERTIES OF CULTURAL SCHEMAS

The implicit message from mothers to daughters that adolescent pregnancy is or is not a desired outcome is in actuality a complex interaction of component messages and emotional attitudes—some communicating educational information and others communicating mothers' beliefs, expectations about daughters' activities, and mothers' implicit intentions and evaluations of their own capabilities influencing the course of daughters' adolescent sexuality. What communicates the desirability or undesirability of adolescent pregnancy from mothers' perspectives is not so much the content of these individual component messages and attitudes, but the context in which they are communicated. For each of the components just described, any given content in the context of a consistent pattern can convey the message that mother is opposed to daughter's potential or actual adolescent pregnancy, whereas the same content in the context of an inconsistent pattern can convey the opposite meaning.

Educational Information

One thing that most daughters learn from mothers, regardless of whether they are given specific detailed information about how babies are made or about how the making of babies can be prevented, is that a girl can get pregnant if she is around boys and does not keep her dress down. The numbers and narratives just presented indicate that virtually all mothers' conscious reasons for teaching daughters this basic fact is to alert them to the dangers of boys and help them to avoid pregnancy. However, for some mothers, another less conscious reason is to provide daughters with information they can utilize in the service of becoming pregnant.

In general, mothers in our sample gave two kinds of educational information to daughters. One pertained to the biological facts of sex, pregnancy, and birth control. The other pertained to the facts of life in the streets—when, where, and under what circumstances girls are most likely to run into boys with single-minded intentions. The latter information was conveyed most often in the context of warning daughters and imposing restrictions on their activities in the streets.

Some mothers (e.g., the mother selected to illustrate the consistent, restrictive, informative schema in the preceding section) conveyed both kinds of information to daughters in the strongest emotional terms. These mothers came across as wanting daughters to know about the dangers and how to avoid them. Other mothers with inconsistent schemas were more selective in giving information, most often regaling daughters with details about life in the streets in an emotionally charged manner, while adopting an attitude of disengagement from daughters that seemed out of keeping with the dangerous picture they themselves constructed. These mothers maintained a distant attitude toward daughters in the joint-interview session, sometimes conveying an undercurrent of anger and hostility, while insisting to interviewers that daughters were not doing anything and therefore did not need detailed information about how to protect themselves from dangers in the streets. This incongruous combination of words, deeds, and emotions created the subjective impression that mothers implicitly condoned and encouraged adolescent sexuality and pregnancy and that detailed information was intended to educate daughters in the process whereby these events could happen. The message communicated by mothers most loudly and clearly, then, depended on the combination of what they said and did, what they did not say or do, and the emotional undertones of both.

Mothers' Beliefs

Mothers' beliefs that birth control pills are harmful in many and varied ways and ineffective in preventing pregnancy are widespread in this population. These beliefs are held by mothers who not only have constructed inconsistent schemas, but also are consistent in their efforts to deter daughters' adolescent pregnancies and are consistent in their attitudes that daughters will take their own prudent steps to avoid this occurrence.

Mothers' beliefs that birth control pills are harmful and ineffectual enter into the communication of double messages when combined with inactivity regarding the giving of information or putting daughters on birth control in the face of suspicions, fears, or actual evidence that daughters are engaging in risky sexual activities. Mothers with inconsistent schemas use these beliefs regarding birth control as justifications to themselves and to others for not taking the steps needed to avoid a consciously unwanted pregnancy. In contrast, mothers with consistent schemas who hold the same beliefs and who may have used this rationalization with regard to their own pregnancies are reluctant to act on those beliefs when faced with the potential pregnancies of their daughters.

This observation regarding mothers' beliefs regarding birth control pills argues against the efficacy of straightforward educational or information-giving intervention programs. Mothers in this community know about birth control pills, know how they work and how they should be taken, and know where to get them, but believe that they have various ill-effects on the functionings of their bodies or minds and/or believe that they do not work for all people (themselves and their daughters, in particular). Inasmuch as these beliefs do not derive from lack of information, the giving of information is unlikely to change them.

Mothers' Expectations About Daughters' Sexual Activities

Mothers have many and varied ways of communicating to daughters their expectations regarding daughters' sexual activities. These communications—sometimes subtle and sometimes not so subtle—convey what mothers fear, believe, or hope daughters are doing in the present or will be doing in the future. Again, whether these communications are interpreted as fears, beliefs, or hopes by daughters or by interviewers is a function of the overall context in which they are expressed.

One way that mothers communicate expectations, for example, is through verbal statements indicating what they expect their daughters or other girls to do. Many mothers tell daughters that when they reach a certain age (usually 16 or 17), they should be apprised of the facts of sex, pregnancy, and other matters because this is the age when girls begin to think about and engage in sexual activities. Many mothers state that they do not tell their daughters about or do not insist that they take birth control pills because the telling or the doing will be interpreted by daughters as license for sexual activity. Many mothers ask daughters if they feel the need to be on birth control pills, thus communicating their expectation that daughter is sexually active. Many mothers tell daughters to come to them first when they feel the desire to be sexually active, when they get that "little love feeling." Some mothers communicate to daughters the expectation that daughters will soon begin dating or "talking to" boys in general or to a specific boy in particular. In the context of consistent presentations, these statements carry the connotation of reality descriptions. In the context of inconsistent presentations, they carry the connotation of hoped-for events.

A second way in which expectations are communicated is through mothers' adversarial or accusatory stances toward daughters regarding their potential sexual activities. Given the proper context, mothers' repeated insistence that daughters are "doing something," regardless of whether daughters are in fact doing anything, can communicate the message that mother is desirous that daughter is doing something.

Mothers' Capabilities

Mothers also have many ways of making known what they can or cannot do with regard to daughters' sexual activities or prospective pregnancies. One of these ways is through mothers' verbal statements and emotional attitudes connoting an incapacity to control daughters' sexual activities, suggesting that daughters will become pregnant if they wish to. Many mothers tell daughters that if they want to have sex, they (mothers) will be unable to stop them; that if daughters want to go out in the streets, they will be unable to tie them to the house; that although daughters are not allowed to entertain boyfriends in their own houses, there is nothing mothers can do to prevent meetings with boys in other people's houses; that they cannot be vigilant all of the time; and that they cannot combat daughters' willfulness and incorrigibility. In the context of consistent presentations, the balance of meaning conveyed by these verbal statements and emotional attitudes is tilted toward a description of reality; That is, statements tend to convey a recognition by mother that the world really is a dangerous place for poor, African American adolescent girls and that if daughters really are determined to get pregnant, they will find a way. In the context of inconsistent presentations, these same statements and attitudes communicate a different meaning—that mother will not impede daughter's progress toward the state of becoming an unwed adolescent mother.

The same ambiguity of meaning applies to other ways in which mothers make known their capabilities or lack thereof regarding daughters' adolescent sexuality. Some of these include mothers' actions in facilitating daughters' activities with boys—arranging meetings, implicitly instructing boys to "talk" to daughters by repeatedly telling them not to, allowing boys to visit daughters at home, not imposing curfews or restrictions on daughters' activities, and the like. Other ways include mothers' verbal statements letting daughters know what to expect if they succeed in becoming pregnant—that daughters will remain pregnant until the baby is born and that they, the mothers, will assist in the raising of the babies. Whether such communications convey a sense of mothers' deep convictions regarding the value of human life and concern for the raising of children or a sense of mothers' hopes for the opportunity to raise their adolescent daughters' children depends on the consistency of mothers' total constellations of statements, actions, and emotional attitudes.

In sum, this analysis of mothers' cultural schemas regarding daughters' adolescent sexuality confirms our previous hypothesis that although virtually all mothers' cultural schemas represent adolescent pregnancy as an unwanted event on a conscious, explicit level, some mothers' schemas represent adolescent pregnancy as an implicit goal at a less conscious level. Amidst variations in the particular configurations of component messages and attitudes constituting schemas, the underlying dimension communicating whether mothers mean what they explicitly say, or also mean the opposite, is consistency. In the context of consistent schemas, component messages and attitudes come across as relatively straightforward and believable descriptions of mothers' conscious realities. In the context of inconsistent schemas, component messages and attitudes connote more than they appear to mean on the surface, and these additional unconscious meanings are the opposite of what is consciously meant on the surface. Mothers' minds, it seems, are exquisitely equipped to communicate what they mean, regardless of whether they consciously know what they mean; daughters' minds are just as equipped to receive what mothers' mean, regardless of whether they consciously know what they have received.

FAMILY CONTEXTS, CULTURAL SCHEMAS, AND ADOLESCENT PREGNANCY STATUS

Relations Among Family Contexts, Cultural Schemas, and Pregnancy

Several important questions can be addressed: How do family environments, cultural schemas, and adolescent pregnancy outcomes for mothers and daughters fit together in our sample? Does growing up in a particular type family environment make it more likely that a woman will establish that type of family environment for her daughter? Is it the case in the larger sample, as among families in the ethnographic phase, that mothers growing up in downwardly mobile or traditional families, or that mothers who themselves were adolescent mothers, are more likely than other mothers to communicate mixed messages to daughters about their sexuality and pregnancy? Are mothers who have grown up in or currently live in downwardly mobile or traditional family environments, who themselves were adolescent mothers or who communicate mixed messages to daughters, more likely than other mothers to have daughters who have become pregnant as adolescents?

Answers to these questions as they pertain to the larger sample can be inferred from Figure 5-1.[3] Contrary to what some might expect, mothers growing up in particular types of family environments in our sample have not necessarily established the same kinds of environments for their daughters, and mothers who themselves were pregnant as adolescents have not necessarily begotten daughters who have become pregnant as adolescents. Furthermore, whether mothers or daughters in this sample have become pregnant as teenagers is not a function of the kinds of family environments in which they have been reared.

However, both the kind of family environment in which a mother grew up and her adolescent pregnancy history have made a difference with regard to the kind of schema she has formed about her daughter's

---

[3] To address questions regarding relations among family environments, cultural schemas, and adolescent pregnancy, we used a statistical procedure appropriate for analyzing categorical data know as loglinear analysis. Generally speaking, loglinear analyses search for a model that best fits the observed relations among two or more categorical variables. Once the model is selected, substantive descriptions of findings from loglinear analyses can be expressed in terms of odds, a ratio of frequencies of a given outcome expected under the "best fit" model to the expected frequencies of other possible outcomes. A technical description of this procedure, the design of the specific analysis conducted, and the statistical results obtained from it are described in Appendix C, section C (1 and 2).

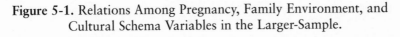

Figure 5-1. Relations Among Pregnancy, Family Environment, and Cultural Schema Variables in the Larger-Sample.

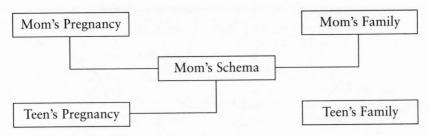

adolescent sexuality, which in turn has made a difference with regard to whether her daughter has become pregnant as an unwed teenager.

To elaborate these findings in more detail,[4] in all three family contexts mothers who were pregnant as adolescents have more often constructed inconsistent schemas than those who were not. Further, regardless of their adolescent pregnancy histories, mothers growing up in downwardly mobile and traditional families have been more likely to construct inconsistent cultural schemas than those growing up in upwardly mobile environments. In the upwardly mobile family context, mothers' adolescent pregnancy histories have made a difference in whether consistent cultural schemas are of the restrictive and informative or nonrestrictive and noninformative type. Former adolescent mothers have been more likely to construct consistent schemas of the restrictive and informative type, and mothers who were not pregnant as adolescents have been more likely to construct schemas of the nonrestrictive and noninformative type. One could say, therefore, that the effects of family environments and pregnancy histories on mothers' cultural schemas have been both compounding and interacting.

As seen in Table 5-2, the odds of being a pregnant adolescent were more than twice as high for daughters of mothers with inconsistent schemas than for daughters of mothers with consistent, restrictive and informative schemas and nine times higher than for daughters of mothers with consistent, nonrestrictive and noninformative schemas.

Although odds were against daughters' adolescent pregnancies for mothers with both kinds of consistent schemas, these numbers indicate that odds of daughters' pregnancies were higher if mothers were consistently active in attempting to prevent them (consistent: restrictive and informative) than if they took a consistently less active role in giving

---

[4] Odds of mothers' cultural schemas are shown in Table C-3, Appendix C, section C (2) as a function of mothers' family environments and adolescent pregnancy status.

Table 5-2. Odds of Daughter's Pregnancy Status Given Mothers'
Cultural Schemas, and Vice Versa

	Mother's Cultural Schema		
	Inconsistent	Consistent	Consistent
		Restrict/Inform	NoRestrict/ NoInform
Daughter's Pregnancy			
Pregnant	1.80/2.70	.87/.23	.21/.09
Not Pregnant	.56/.68	1.14/.28	4.67/.61

Note. Numbers on left side of slash (/) are the odds of daughter's pregnancy status given mother's cultural schema classification. Numbers on right side are odds of mother's cultural schema classification given daughter's pregnancy status. Odds are a ratio of expected frequencies of a given outcome under the best fit model to the expected frequencies of other possible outcomes. For example, the odds are 1.80 to 1 under the best fit model that daughter will be in the Pregnant category given an inconsistent mother schema; conversely the odds are 2.70 to 1 that mother's schema will be inconsistent given a daughter in the Pregnant category. Restrict/Inform = restrictive and informative; NoRestrict/NoInform = nonrestrictive and noninformative.

information or setting rules (consistent: nonrestrictive and noninformative). The possibility that the fact of daughters' pregnancy status might account for differences in levels of activity reflected in mothers' consistent schemas was rejected on two empirical grounds. First, the odds for both kinds of consistent schemas for mothers of pregnant daughters were quite low, both in the absolute sense and in relation to the odds of inconsistent schemas. Second, when mothers' schemas were used to predict daughters' pregnancy outcomes, prediction error was reduced by 33%; conversely, when daughters' pregnancy status was used to predict mothers' schemas, no reduction (0%) of error was achieved.[5]

Demographic Correlates of Family Environments, Cultural Schemas, and Adolescent Pregnancy Status

Two demographic variables that were not used in constructing family environment categories were current family income and total numbers of years of formal education completed by mothers. Although all families selected for this study were poor, as determined by their eligibility for the free-lunch program, we thought it possible that variations in income levels

---

[5] This estimate of the reduction of error when values of one variable are used to predict the values of the other was based on the Goodman–Kruskal measure of predictability. If this particular type of association is absent, $\lambda = 0$. If the independent variable perfectly specifies the categories of the dependent variable, $\lambda = 1$.

within this narrow range could be directly or indirectly associated with adolescent pregnancy outcomes. Further, although daughters did not differ with respect to levels of educational attainment (i.e., virtually all were currently attending high school), mothers of daughters varied with respect to the total numbers of years of formal education. We thought it possible that mothers' educational levels could be associated with the kinds of current family environments or cultural schemas they have constructed, and with adolescent pregnancy outcomes for themselves or their daughters.[6]

Current family income. Mothers' and teens' current family income levels were not directly associated with adolescent pregnancy histories for mothers or teens or with mothers' cultural schemas—the only variable shown in the previous analysis to be directly associated with daughters' adolescent pregnancy outcomes. An association was found, however, between families' current income levels and current family environment classifications. Families that are currently downwardly mobile earn significantly less on the average than those that are currently either traditional or upwardly mobile. This difference reflects the relatively greater percentages of downwardly mobile single-parent households and downwardly mobile households with no adult employed full time (cf. Table B-3, Appendix B (B-2). Similar head of household and employment patterns for mothers' families of origin would suggest a similar income differential for those as well, although mothers were unable to give us sufficient information about income levels for their families of origin to confirm or disconfirm this hypothesis.

The numbers in Table C-4, Appendix C indicate, however, that whereas mothers' current family incomes are related to current family environments (labeled "Teen's Family" in the table), they are unrelated to the kinds of family environments in which mothers grew up (labeled "Mother's Family" in the table). Thus, growing up in a downwardly mobile family does not doom a woman in this population to greater poverty as an adult than growing up in a traditional or upwardly mobile family; conversely, growing up in an upwardly mobile family is not a guarantee of greater prosperity relative to women growing up in traditional or downwardly mobile family environments.

Mothers' educational levels. Direct associations were observed in this sample between mothers' educational levels and their adolescent pregnancy histories. One can interpret the relation between mothers' educational levels and their adolescent pregnancy histories in various ways. Dropping out of school may predispose a girl toward an adolescent

---

[6] The relevant data are shown in Table C-4, Appendix C, section C (3).

pregnancy, an adolescent pregnancy may cut an educational career short, or girls with certain personal characteristics may be more likely than others to stay in school and delay pregnancy. These are all likely to be true. Teens in our sample, however, were attending high school at the time. Those who had become pregnant did so while attending school and returned to school following the child's birth, leaving the baby in the care of mother. Although it is likely that those teens who had babies at the time of our interviews will end up completing fewer years of formal education than those who did not have babies at the time of our interviews, it can be said with certainty that, for this teen sample, school attendance was not a factor differentiating those who had or had not become pregnant as teenagers.

Mothers' educational levels and their cultural schemas were also significantly associated. One can surmise that mothers who themselves were able to stay in school and delay pregnancy beyond the teenage years believe that the same can be possible for their daughters, despite evidence and messages to the contrary that may be all around them in their social environments.

Cultural Schemas in Context

Strictly speaking, the immediate reasons why some teenage girls in our sample have become unwed mothers are not because they are poor, because they have grown up in downwardly mobile family environments, because they are from single-parent homes, because they or their mothers have been or are on welfare, or because their own mothers were pregnant as adolescents; girls have not become pregnant because they are ignorant of sex, pregnancy, or birth control or because they lack access to contraceptives. All of the mother–daughter dyads in this study were poor, and neither variations of income within the sample nor qualitative structural and extended-kin networking characteristics of families related directly to mothers' or daughters' adolescent pregnancy status. More immediately, the results of this study thus far suggest that some poor, African American adolescent girls in this region become pregnant because their mothers communicate explicit messages that birth control pills are harmful and implicit messages that adolescent pregnancies outside of marriage are desirable and because daughters internalize mothers' messages as prescriptions for action.

In this sample, it is not the sociocultural context per se that differentiates girls who have or have not become pregnant as teenagers, but rather the manner in which mothers and daughters have cognitively and emotionally construed the desirability or undesirability of adolescent pregnancies within that context. The impact of mothers' family-of-origin environments and mothers' own adolescent histories on daughters' adolescent pregnancy outcomes is filtered through channels internal to the minds of both mothers and daughters.

Yet, at the same time that adolescent pregnancy outcomes are more directly tied to internal meanings than contexts, meanings cannot be constructed, communicated, or interpreted outside of contexts. It is through analysis of contexts that meanings, especially deeper ones, are revealed. For example, only in an historical context can we understand the importance of extended-kin networking in this population and the pressures that have required contemporary families to abandon or modify this strategy for survival in the face of continuing oppression and scarcity. As discussed in chapters 2 and 3, networking has served vital functions, albeit changing ones, for African Americans since precolonial West African times.

Similarly, conclusions drawn in the previous section regarding family income and educational attainments must be placed in the context of two facts: one, that all of the families in our sample were poor, and two, that all of the teenage girls were attending high school. It is possible and indeed probable that statistical associations between income levels and the family environment, cultural schema, and adolescent pregnancy variables examined in this chapter would be significant in a sample that included families from all levels of the income spectrum. It is also likely that teenage pregnancy rates in the population sampled in the study are higher among those girls who have dropped out of school than among those who have not. Our data show, however, that when these conditions are held constant to a great degree, variations still occur in pregnancy outcomes. Although poverty may provide nourishment for the seeds of adolescent pregnancy, some seeds grow in the soil of poverty and others do not. Conversely, whereas school attendance and higher levels of education may contribute to an environment that is unfriendly toward adolescent pregnancy, some seeds still take root in this environment.

Another way that context makes a difference is with regard to the meanings daughters attribute to mothers' words, deeds, and emotions. In the context of inconsistencies among these various manifestations of mothers' schemas, the explicit meanings of mothers' words clash with implicit meanings, signifying ambivalence and contradiction in mothers' attitudes about daughters' adolescent sexuality. In the context of consistent presentations by mothers, explicit and implicit meanings coincide. The data from this sample indicate that implicit meanings in mothers' schemas are most closely related to daughters' adolescent pregnancy outcomes.

A narrow focus on mothers with inconsistent schemas alone might lend credence to an argument that daughters of these mothers become pregnant because of lack of restrictions or information about sex, pregnancy, and contraception. Mothers in this population, it could be said, are ill-equipped or unsupported in their attempts to accomplish the two essential tasks of educating daughters or setting enforceable limits. A broader focus on both inconsistent and consistent schemas, however, makes clear that this interpretation holds little water. Mothers least likely to have ever-pregnant daughters portrayed themselves as disinclined toward both specific information-giving and rule-setting. When viewed within this context, it is neither mothers' information-giving nor rule-setting per se that makes the difference in daughters' eventual adolescent pregnancy status, but rather mothers' deeply held and mostly unconscious convictions that adolescent pregnancy is or is not the desired path for daughters to take.

Context is also critical in understanding the basis of mothers' implicit beliefs that adolescent pregnancy is a desirable outcome. On the face of it, the idea that some mothers want their daughters to become pregnant at any mental level seems to contradict the assumption that mothers generally want what is best for their daughters and, for some readers, may imply a "blame-the-victim" perspective. As our empirical data have shown, however, mothers' cultural schemas have been constructed within and at least partly reflect pressures emanating from their own family-of-origin environments, educational experiences, and adolescent pregnancy histories. Within these contexts, mothers' implicit beliefs can be understood as being in the best interest of their daughters. Mothers with certain past experiences—especially mothers with less education who gave birth as adolescents and themselves have grown up in downwardly mobile or traditional family environments—hedge their bets with regard to daughters' chances for achieving the middle-class American dream, betting most of their money, so to speak, on the probability that daughters' well-being will best be served by establishing networks of social and economic exchange. For these mothers, we speculate that implicit messages promoting adolescent pregnancy are motivated by hierarchical schemas in which adolescent pregnancy is an intermediate goal along the way to the establishment and maintenance of networks—the latter constituting the superordinate goal of "success."

In contrast, mothers who grew up in upwardly mobile environments believe that daughters can achieve the middle-class dream—the superordinate goal in these mothers' success schemas. Further, upwardly mobile mothers rely on their own past adolescent histories to determine how much trust to place in daughters to make the right choices along the way versus how much they as disciplinarians and educators need to actively intervene in matters relating to daughters' adolescent sexuality. Upwardly mobile mothers who were themselves able to delay pregnancy and who themselves may have achieved higher levels of education than other mothers are more likely than other mothers to construct consistent schemas in which adolescent pregnancy is an impediment to personal and socioeconomic growth and in which daughters are endowed with the capacity of self-determination, of making these growth producing choices on their own, just as mothers themselves were able to make these choices. What is most important in our findings is that it is not mothers' life experiences themselves that make the difference with regard to daughters' pregnancy outcomes, but rather the ways in which these experiences have been translated by mothers into representations and beliefs about daughters' potentialities.

6

Internal Working Models of Attachment in the Adolescent Pregnancy System

A further context within which adolescent pregnancy in this poor African American population takes on meaning is the mother–daughter relationship. What mothers and daughters in the ethnographic phase said about their relationships with each other seemed linked in comprehensible ways to their thoughts, feelings, and behavior regarding adolescent pregnancy. In designing the larger-sample interview phase, therefore, we looked for a measure that could capture the essence of respondents' representations of these relationships. As was the case in our investigation of sociocultural variables discussed in the previous chapter, the first questions asked with regard to mother–daughter relationships were whether the same constellations of characteristics discovered in the ethnographic phase (e.g., the deprived and competitive working models) adequately characterize the mothers and daughters in the larger sample, whether modifications of or additions to these earlier descriptions are in order, and whether entirely different descriptions are needed.

The AAI (George et al., 1985) suited our needs in the larger-sample phase of the study because it focused on individuals' mental representations of their past and current relationships with parents and other significant attachment figures, it allowed for the presentation of a standard set of questions to a larger number of adolescent girls and their mothers, and it permitted flexibility on the parts of interviewers and respondents in elaborating on and clarifying questions and responses.

The AAI suited our purposes but, as we discussed in chapter 4, the procedures developed by Main and her colleagues for coding interviews did not. These procedures focus more on quality of thought, or the manner in which respondents approach the discussion of attachment-related issues, than on the content of what they say about their relationships.

Although both components enter into Main's coding scheme, quality of thought more so than content determines the ultimate classifications of respondents as secure, insecure (preoccupied, dismissing), or disorganized. By relegating content to the back burner, so to speak, Main's scheme does not capture two properties of internal working models we suspect are important in the adolescent pregnancy system: predominant themes in respondents' representations of relationships (e.g., deprivation, competition) and levels of structural differentiation within representations of goals, fears, defensive strategies, and persons or person roles.

With regard to themes, quality of thought does not capture respondents' specific, unconscious, person-related goals; their characteristic modalities for attempting to accomplish goals; their specific fantasied or expected consequences or outcomes of such attempts; and the specific deeper level defensive maneuvers by which respondents attempt to reconcile desired goals with external reality and their judgments of what is prudent, acceptable, or allowable by self and others. With regard to structural differentiation of persons or person roles, quality of thought does not capture respondents' unconscious perspectives on differences between mother and father roles or functions in relationships, on differences between their own thoughts or feelings and those of others, or on the possibilities that others (mothers and fathers) can have relationships that do not include them. These thematic and structural properties were identifiable in the talk of women in the ethnographic phase and seemed linked more than quality of thought to women's adolescent pregnancy histories. Further, whereas thematic or structural properties of women's working models appeared to remain stable over the 3-year period of our ethnographic research, women's quality of thought when conversing with us about relationship issues did not.

To illustrate, we return again to the excerpts of interviews with Yolanda, Lynetta, Aretha, and Rachel reported in chapter 3. Both Yolanda and Lynetta, as these excerpts suggest, wished for a closer, intimate relationship with their mothers but expected or believed that their mothers did not wish for such a relationship with them. The overriding feelings engendered by these women's talk about their relationships were those of rejection and emotional deprivation. To protect against these feelings, both women had mobilized unconscious defenses that were only partially successful in warding off the associated anxiety. Lynetta, for example, asserted that she did not wish to be a mother because her own parents did not want to be adults—"They're wishing they was a child." At the same time, however, she knew her parents "love taking care of (her)." In these comments we can hear Lynetta's wish to be loved by mother, her unconscious representation of mother as not wanting to be a mother (an adult), and her defensive competing and more conscious representation of mother as loving. The inadequacy of this latter defense, however, was manifested by Lynetta's subsequent comment that she wished to give her mother something to remember her by when she grew up. Implied in this statement is the continuing representation of mother as rejecting (i.e., mother would require a gift in order to remember her) and the anticipation of defensive action that might forestall the expected, unwelcomed outcome of mother not remembering her (i.e., giving her mother a gift).

Similarly, Yolanda's descriptions of her relationship with her own mother were filled with contradictory representations and clear defensive maneuvers for avoiding anxiety. One statement—"She had to have loved me if she took care of me and I was that bad"—condenses both rejecting and loving representations of mother and reflects her defensive strategies of first turning angry feelings toward the "rejecting" mother against herself and then rationalizing that a mother who would put up with such a bad child must be doing it out of love. Thus Yolanda transforms the rejecting mother into the good mother by making herself into the bad child—a solution that may alleviate but not overcome her anxiety.

In talking to us about her relationships, Lynetta exhibited a quality of thought that can best be described as preoccupied. As time went on, this quality of thought became increasingly disorganized. In our later interviews when she was 16, Lynetta spoke in a highly agitated fashion without interruption for many minutes at a time, regaling us with minute details of only tangentially related thoughts, feelings, and experiences. In contrast, Yolanda presented herself initially as dismissing. When we first met her, Yolanda claimed to remember very little about her childhood relationships with mother, father, or siblings, choosing to talk about them if at all in overly generalized, unconvincing, idealized terms. In our early conversations, such as the one reported in chapter 3, she spoke of her parents in ways that admitted no fault; denied knowledge of any details of her parents' lives, stating that if we wanted to know we should ask them; and professed to have no idea or concern regarding the current activities or whereabouts of her numerous brothers and stepbrothers. She guessed they were "just out doing what people do." Later, however, Yolanda remembered a lot more about her parents and siblings, which she was able to discuss in a much more thoughtful and reflective manner. She acknowledged that her parents in fact had not been good parents—that her father had abused her mother and herself, her mother had been uninvolved and ineffectual and had ultimately abandoned her and her siblings—and reflected that her parents' own lives had been very difficult (i.e., her father had been laid off and the family left with no source of income and all four grandparents had died at young ages, leaving the family without a support system). She confessed that when we had first asked her these questions, she had felt they were none of our business, that she had no reason to trust us, and that she was concerned about what we might think. This more reflective and insightful way of talking about her childhood, however, neither changed Yolanda's underlying representation of it as depriving nor diluted Yolanda's regret and feelings of anger, resentment, and sadness that she had not and still did not have a close relationship with her mother.

Aretha's and Rachel's internal working models proper, in contrast to Yolanda's and Lynetta's, represented mothers (or grandmothers) as hostile, threatening figures bent on interfering with their relationships with men (fathers, stepfathers, boyfriends). Implied in these representations are Aretha's and Rachel's wishes to have a special relationship with father (or father substitute) that excludes mother. To defend against the anxiety associated with the prospect of mother's retaliation for such a wish—a prospect made all the more real by mothers' physically and verbally aggressive behavior toward Rachel and Aretha—both girls adopted conciliatory attitudes toward mother, Rachel's manifesting itself in the forms of expressions of unqualified devotion and a moral prohibition against being disrespectful toward mother, and Aretha's in the form of remaining close and sharing her valued possessions (including her infants) with grandmother. In speaking to us about these matters, Aretha from the start was open about her feelings and exhibited a flexible and insightful quality of thought. She hoped that her experiences with Martha would help her create a different environment for her own daughter's development. Rachel initially presented herself as highly preoccupied, but later talked about her relationships in a more moderated, insightful, and resigned manner.

These examples from our ethnographic observations indicate (a) that there are several sources of variation among internal working models, only one of which is an individual's quality of thought in reflecting on or talking about them and (b) that quality of thought, although reflecting individuals' feelings of security or insecurity about these represented relationships, may not bear a one-to-one correspondence to these other sources of variation. A further point highlighted by these descriptions is that the anxiety associated with reflections and discourse about internal working models may lessen or increase as an individual approaches certain sensitive topics, or develops a more familiar relationship with an interviewer, with the consequence that the individual's quality of thought in discussing relationships with that interviewer may change.

This observation, I believe, is consistent with Main's (1995) description of organized insecure attachment categories (preoccupied, dismissing) as "transference-like patterns of interaction between interviewer and interviewee" (p. 443). In a psychoanalysis, an analysand's characteristic ways of protecting herself from anticipated dangers in relationships are routinely adopted or transferred in the developing, intrapsychic relationship with the analyst. As the working alliance between analysand and analyst develops and deepens, and as analysis proceeds, these defenses may be recognized as maladaptive and given up in favor of others that allow for a less guarded and more satisfactory expression of thoughts and feelings. A similar phenomenon may be at work in a developing, ongoing relationship between a researcher and research participants. If that is the case, then we would expect the other, perhaps more stable sources of variation represented in internal working models proper to provide a better indication of the underlying "security" of an attachment relationship than quality of thought.

Given these considerations, we adopted a method for coding the AAI that differentiated mothers and daughters with respect to quality of thought and content. The technical details of this method are described in detail in chapter 4 and Appendix A. For both quality of thought and internal working models proper, our method proceeded in two complementary directions simultaneously: one toward the discovery of meaning and the other toward the identification of patterns that signify meanings.

The task of identifying meaningful patterns in mothers' and daughters' representations of attachment relationships, both quality-of-thought and internal working model proper components, was similar in some ways but different in others from the identification and interpretation of patterns signifying cultural schemas. It was similar in that meanings were used to recognize patterns and patterns were used to verify and elaborate meanings as well as to classify particular individuals as repositories of particular meanings.

It was different in that we brought considerably more theoretical baggage with us to the task. Whereas the general concept of culturally constituted cognitive schemas fits into an emerging theoretical framework constructed by cultural psychologists and anthropologists (e.g., D'Andrade, 1990), schemas themselves are by definition culture specific and issue specific. They are representations of specific hierarchies of goals, actions, and actors within specific cultures that may or may not have relevance to other issues or other cultures. The meanings we eventually attributed to the four cultural schemas identified in chapter 5 and our analyses of ways in which mothers communicate two different messages simultaneously were derived directly from women's narratives and not from a preexisting theoretical framework.

In contrast, although labeled differently, the constructs termed internal working models proper and quality of thought in this chapter have been identified and discussed by numerous theorists of varied persuasions in relation to individuals from assorted cultures and socioeconomic groups. To name just some of these preexisting theoretical contexts, similar constructs have been conceptualized within the frameworks of attachment theory (e.g., Bowlby, 1973; Bretherton, 1985, 1990, 1991; Main et al., 1985), event representation theory (e.g., Bretherton, 1985, 1990, 1991; Nelson, 1983), and psychoanalysis (e.g., Erikson, 1963; Loewald, 1980; Sandler & Rosenblatt, 1962). Whereas some of the particulars and the labels we have assigned these models may be unique, their properties as discerned through qualitative analyses of narratives are familiar enough to identify them as belonging in the same general domain as models, schemas, intrapsychic structures, and processes talked about by many others.

The task of identifying patterns and meanings can be facilitated by overlap with preexisting theoretical perspectives. The more one knows about something, the easier it is to find it, and the more meaning can be attributed to it once it is found. We acknowledge, however, that at the same time that prior knowledge of patterns and processes facilitates finding and understanding them, it can also obscure discovery of other possible patterns and processes. The very facts that cluster analyses of principal component scores can produce numerous sets of patterns from the same data and people looking at these various patterns through different theoretical lenses can attribute different meanings leave open the possibility that the cluster solutions we have chosen and the interpretations we will make may not be the only possible ways of understanding mothers' and daughters' representations.

With this caveat in mind, we proceed to qualitative descriptions and illustrations of characteristics of quality-of-thought and internal working model proper classifications as we have constructed them from our data and to quantitative analyses of relations among these "personal" representational variables and with adolescent pregnancy outcomes. In this chapter and the next, we examine alternative theoretical frameworks that can comprehend these characteristics for better or for worse.

QUALITY OF THOUGHT

The quality-of-thought characteristics of women identified through qualitative analyses in our study were quite similar to those described for secure, preoccupied, and dismissing classifications in other studies using the AAI (Fonagy, Steele, & Steele, 1991; Haft & Slade, 1989; Kobak et al., 1989; Main & Goldwyn, in press). These characteristics are summarized in Table 6-1.

Table 6-1. Quality-of-Thought Categories for Teens and Mothers

Preoccupied: Preoccupied respondents do not consistently maintain a focus on the topic at hand. They give the impression through an overabundance of verbal output, vacillations between favorable versus unfavorable descriptions of attachment figures and relationships, and an overtly angry or frenetic tone, of still struggling with childhood attachment-related conflicts and feelings. Detailed memories may be reported, but they may have inconsistent implications that are not integrated into a coherent picture. As a result, the interview may seem difficult to follow.

Dismissing: Dismissing respondents maintain a focus on the topic but convey their responses with passivity and resistance. Dismissing respondents remember few of their childhood experiences and downplay the significance of experiences for current functioning. Thoughts about past lives and relationships are often separated from feelings.

Secure: Secure respondents maintain a focus on the topic and convey their responses in an open, objective, thoughtful, coherent, and affectively appropriate manner. Respondents demonstrate insight about attachment relationships and regard them as influential in the development of their current personalities. Seemingly contradictory memories can be integrated into a coherent and believable picture.

INTERNAL WORKING MODELS PROPER

Teen and Mother–Mother Interviews

Table 6-2 describes the characteristics of the three main categories of internal working models proper derived through qualitative analyses for the teen and mother–mother interviews. As described in chapters 3 and 4, three main categories of the internal working model proper variable (deprived, competitive, and mature) were each subdivided into two (deprived–acknowledged and deprived–denied; competitive–acknowledged and competitive–denied; mature, father–distant and mature, father–close), with the exception that only one competitive category was derived for teens. In the following descriptions, characteristics described pertain to both subcategories of a given main category except where subcategories are specifically distinguished.

Table 6-2. Internal Working Model Proper Categories for Teens and Mothers

Deprived

Respondents in this category emphasize themes of emotional and/or material deprivation in their relationships with both parents. Past struggles and desires to elicit or obtain parental affection, attention, or material goods are described with anger, yearning, and wistfulness. Rivalries abound with siblings, stepparents, or other categories of parents' friends for attention and special treatment by mother or father.

Relationships depicted in these interviews are predominantly dyadic and more undifferentiated relative to other models with regard to representations of parents, parental roles, and self–other distinctions. Respondents describe wanting similar things from both parents (material goods, attention, caring, closeness) and describe both mothers and fathers as potential providers of these wants. Descriptions of a relationship between mother and father that is separate and distinct from either the mother–daughter or father–daughter relationship are notably absent. Blurring of boundaries between self and others is manifested in the fluidity with which respondents shift between their own and their parents' perspectives, in confusions about child versus parental roles, and in confusions about perpetrator–victim roles.

In deprived–acknowledged interviews, themes of emotional and material deprivation are relatively less disguised by defensive maneuvers than in deprived–denied interviews, with themes framed in context of open conflict, intrigue, deception, suspiciousness, defiance, and violence. Defensive tactics in both kinds of deprived interviews, however, include overidealizations; turning negative to positive; stressing the satisfactions of the caretaking role rather than of being cared for; using the absence of negative events to support characterization of the relationship as positive; identifying with mother's criticisms; and denial of the negative impact of parental abuse, rejection, or neglect.

Competitive

Representations of mothers in childhood by competitive respondents are as harsh, critical, and often hostile disciplinarians, whereas fathers are depicted as caring, understanding, faithful, and often seductive confidants whose roles are to protect and rescue daughters from mothers. Daughter remembers herself as being Daddy's girl, and as competing with mother for the affections of father. This characterization may apply as well to the present day but more frequently has been replaced by anger and resentment that she (daughter) has been rejected, abandoned, or replaced in father's affections by someone else. Present-day representations of mother may continue as per childhood but more frequently have been replaced by one of mother as a less threatening, more supportive, and even idealized figure who is perceived as having stood by daughter's side in the face of father's infidelity or disappearance.

Competitive representations are by definition triadic and clearly differentiate self from other and mother from father roles.

Mature

Respondent conveys the sense in these interviews of having received needed emotional supplies from her childhood relationship with mother despite possible difficulties or setbacks in that relationship. Mother is described as having fostered progressive development—for example, as having helped daughter to understand life's problems and how to deal with them, helped her to develop confidence in her own ability to become a competent person, and helped her to define goals. Daughter describes herself as having identified with mother's aspirations for her, with mother's way of interacting with people, coping with problems, showing affection or displeasure, and with mother's interests and competencies. A general positive relationship picture may be interspersed with descriptions of mother's inadequacies, failures, or undesirable characteristics, but the latter are depicted as more circumscribed than general in scope and do not dominate the interview.

Respondent's relationship with father is represented by a mature respondent as either incidental and inconsequential in relation to the mother–daughter relationship or as important in both daughter's and mother's worlds. For representations in which fathers play an active role, fathers are valued and appreciated for their dependability, predictability, consistency, faithfulness, tolerance, physical presence, and provider roles more so than for their capacities or interests in understanding or relating to their daughters on an emotional level, the latter qualities being reserved for mothers. Although there may be unfavorable aspects to a respondent's description of father, these do not dominate the interview. Respondents in this category may acknowledge, implicitly or explicitly, that mother and father have or have had a relationship with each other that is all of their own, that is separate from their respective relationships with the children, and that mother values (valued) her relationship with father, whether or not it has been preserved. Thus, structurally, these interviews correspond to those in those in the Competitive category.

Mother–Teen Interviews

Table 6-3 presents descriptions of internal working model proper categories derived through qualitative analyses of the mother–teen interview—the variable that we labeled *mother's representation of daughter's attachment relationships*. As mentioned in chapter 4, cluster analyses identified only two mothers in the Good Mom/Bad Dad category, and thus it was combined with the Bad Mom/Bad Dad category to form The Mixed Mom/Bad Dad category.

Table 6-3. Mother's Representation of Daughter's Attachment Relationship Categories

Group 1: Bad Mom, Bad Dad

In this category, mothers describe their daughters' relationships with themselves and with fathers as fraught with conflict and emotional distance. Daughters' relationships with mothers, however, are depicted as relatively better than with father. Daughters are depicted as incorrigible, especially since adolescence. At best, fathers in these mothers' eyes are worthless and unhelpful, and at worst as violent and threatening. Mothers represent themselves as victimized, helpless, and downtrodden.

Group 2: Bad Mom, Good Dad

In this category, mothers describe their daughters as having been "Daddy's girl" since childhood. This alliance between father and daughter is described in resentful, angry tones. Mother depicts daughter as having a distorted view of her and as being responsible for their tension-filled interactions.

Group 3: Good Mom, Bad Dad

In this category, mothers describe their daughters' relationship with themselves in very positive terms, often verging on overidealization. Fathers in these interviews are denigrated and dismissed as unhelpful or unimportant.

Group 4: Good Mom, Good Dad

In this category, mothers describe their daughters' relationship with both parents as good, despite the acknowledgment that daughters may have preferred or continue to prefer father over mother. Rather than responding to daughter's affection for the fathers in a competitive, resentful way, mothers in this category value and support it. Mothers describe their relationships with fathers and husbands as valued.

EXCERPTS

To illustrate thematic and structural characteristics of internal working model proper categories, excerpts are presented from both mother–mother and teen interviews. Mothers excerpted come from different dyads than teens, and no individual teen or mother interview is excerpted more than once.

Deprived

Teen A. This teen is preoccupied throughout her interview with memories of both mother and father as withholding material goods, much-wanted attention, and emotional supplies. She vacillates between (a) an accusatory stance toward her parents and blaming herself for their angry and rejecting attitudes and (b) memories of wanting to please and wanting to oppose. Memories of feeling close or wishes to be close or to please are routinely followed in this teen's associations by thoughts of parents as rejecting.

She begins the interview with a half-hearted and unconvincing try to reconstruct memories of a warm, close relationship with mother, but she is unable to sustain the effort. Her memories quickly shift to the incessant struggles and fights over material supplies (money) and mother's impossible demands that characterized their relationship:

> I feel really close to my mother, ah, really, because she always, when I just a little baby, she always used to keep me warm and all that . . . and she dress nice . . . and if I ask her to go to town with her, to make groceries, she'll say "You have to sneak off and hide from the little ones," 'cause she won't be liking them going . . . and she always be fussing at me. She didn't want nobody be going to talk to her. When I don't, when I get sleepy, I get hit, I get fussed at. I go, "Yeah, woman." I just say, "Yeah, that woman makes me sick." And I get mad at her when she don't give me things, and you'll take it out of her wallet, or something, she'll get mean and say, "All right, who took it? I know somebody got it. Give me my money." She goes to my purse, look right there, at the money, and go . . . I said, "I'm sorry. I put it in my purse." And she say, "Why you been in my purse?"

Teen remembers her relationship with father in much the same way:

And my Daddy, when he get mad, he tell me to give him some-thing, he'll say "Go buy me a watermelon." I say, "No, I'm not buying nobody nothing. See? I would have to give you my money." I said, "Well, I'm going to buy your watermelon. Which one you want? The big, juicy one? Or the big, skinny, ah, one, that's not juicy?" He said, "Well, give me any one that's cheap." So I brought him back a little sixty-two cent one. He said "I don't want this watermelon." I said, "Well, that mean you spend my money for nothing!"

The issue of who is responsible for these frustrating interactions becomes blurred when teen momentarily turns the blame on herself. This position, however, is quickly reversed by a return to recriminating and denigrating memories of her father's laziness and of herself as having to play the role of disciplinarian:

When I grew up, I always used to spite my Daddy, and he be say-ing "Be quiet, be quiet." And I wouldn't be listening, and he'll say "Be quiet." Go in through one ear, going out the other. And he be lazy. Don't like to get up to do nothing. If he has a little grass that he has to mow, my Mama will bring it outside and put the gas in the mower, and mow the whole yard. When he say, "Come here and light this thing [his cigarette], I say "You too lazy." I say "Go get your lazy self up and get it yourself."

Mother A. This mother approaches the memories of her punitive and withholding mother and father openly. She is clear in her representation of her own mother as denying material things, as denying emotional access, and being unapproachable and even punitive at times of daughter's distress or physical injury:

Let's see, I know when we were smaller we used to catch a lot of whuppings, you know, being bad I guess, getting into devilment. And you know, like whatever we saw the other kids with, we wanted the same thing, but you know they [her parents] wasn't able at the time to get it. And you know, the brothers and the sis-ters would get into a fight and things like that. Then that would be another whipping for us. And when I was going to school, I guess it was a habit or something, I never would associate with anybody, I would be to myself. I never did any talking. And they used to have, I forget what you call them, dovewood switches?

And we would be scared of that because they had little knots on them, and they whip you with that—it be stinging and burning. So we, I always tried to be quiet and I wouldn't catch a whipping. And I remember when my next to oldest sister, she was small and her and my second oldest brother, you know, they was playing and he had a little book he wanted to read and she didn't want him to read it, and she jerk it from him, and he had a little toy gun and she took the little gun from him and cut him on his forehead. So that broke her, my Mama, up from buying them toys, you know, like at Christmas time. During that time, we never did get toys or anything. When I was small, they had these fences that was close to the house and I was climbing and I fell and slit my thigh, you know, wide open on the side, and after I had did it, I was scared you know to tell it and then my mind kept a saying, you better go ahead and tell it and get it over with. If you gonna catch a whipping you might as well, you know, go ahead and get your whipping before the night, you know, so I just goed on and told.

Likewise, this mother's memories of father are of a man who had only two speeds—unresponsive and punitive:

If you ask him something, he would never answer you. Like when I was going to school and I would need, you know, like a quarter, fifty cents, you would ask him, you know he never would answer you. He'd set and look a while, and then he'd just go in his pocket and get it, but never would say, you know, I don't have it or I have it, you know, that's the way he is. We didn't, you know, never say, you know, be around him to make him talk after we see, you know, he wasn't responding back, you know, talking to us, so we always did more associating with our mother than we did with him. We was scared of his whuppings. Once I threw a knife in my older brother's back, and when he come home he whip me and I mean I can remember, you know, that whupping look like it lasted me for two days. Looks like when they started whipping you they whip you so long, they don't know when to stop you know. Like my daddy, he would give you more, about fifteen or sixteen licks . . . I have some nieces and nephews . . . look like they Mama doesn't punish them like, you know, our parents did us.

In this passage, mother struggles with the emotional pain that might be generated by such memories by searching for the good in a mostly bleak picture:

It don't have, you know, any downfalls on me, because you know, I'm glad that, you know, they raised me up like they did because, you know, they kept me out, you know, of getting into trouble.

Teen B. For this teen, themes of emotional and material deprivation are not far beneath the surface of her descriptions of relationships with mother and step-Dad. These themes are thinly disguised by overidealizations and other defenses which are ineffective in preventing memories and thoughts of rejection and deprivation from entering consciousness. Throughout the interview, teen moves back and forth, sometimes within the space of a single sentence, between representations of mother as controlling, demanding, rejecting, and desirous of reversing roles with daughter on the one hand and loving, caring, and solicitous of daughter's feelings on the other. The same vacillation characterizes her representations of step-Dad as caring and generous at the same time that he has absented himself from teen's life altogether. As in the two previous examples, representations of relationships with mother and father and representations of mother and father roles in relationships are qualitatively undifferentiated.

Teen begins with a representation of mother as loving and caring:

Well, well, all I have to say, I'm just, I just was used to being stuck under my Mama a lot. And we didn't you know, know my daddy that well. Me and my mother got along really good. She was nice. She was honest a little bit. I look back on nights when I was small, she took care of me. When my father died, she stay by her room, but she took care of me.

This picture begins to dim as teen remembers having to follow mother's orders, a memory she dispenses with in short order by turning negative to positive:

I guess, when I was young, you know, I gotta, I gotta do what my mother say, she was by me, by my side all the time, she, um, never left me.

A similar transformation occurs in the next sentence, where teen's need blurs into mother's need:

Whenever I needed something, you know, she was, she'll be right in the kitchen, and I just call her, she'll come when I call her. Anything I needed she'll get. Like if she needed, if she had to talk about something, she just sit down and talk to me like, you know, like, if I could, you know, really give her an answer for anything. I hardly didn't know what to do, but she talk to me more or less like she talk to my, you know, (older) sister, I guess.

Teen justifies her picture of mother as caring by thinking of uncaring things mother did not do:

When my father died, you know, she didn't lie to me, and tell me like, she told me that he was my father, you know, she could have told me that her other husband was my father. But when I was small I didn't remember anybody. I go by what she told me.

Teen remembers mother as mean, which she tries to justify on the basis of her own bad behavior, but then she revises the memory to a view of mother as nice:

When I used to pick up stuff or mess with something I had no business with, she get mean, and she keep hollering, you know, telling me the same thing over and over again and I go back and do it again, she get mean! She just, she just get tired of hollering. She was there when I needed to talk, that's all. It was nice, she wasn't mean, she was nice. That's why I like to be with her because she wasn't mean or nothing.

Although teen seemed to be unsure about most other aspects of her representation of mother, she was clear about mother's emotional response to her incipient adolescent sexuality:

When I had to go and buy pads I got embarrassed. I used to take my mother to the store, she was really happy, talking about I was like becoming a young lady.

Step-Dad comes across in this teen's narrative in pretty much the same conflicting light as mother:

My step-Dad, he's nice, he makes our bed, he's like intelligent, you know, like if I ask him if I can get something. He's a sweet person really. [Do you still see him?] Not really, like if I see him, you know, his mother house is in Clearview. Like if I pass through there he probably be outside or something. In the past few years, he would give me anything I wanted. He'll go buy me a bike, if I wanted money, he'll give me money; if I wanted dolls, he'll buy me dolls. We really haven't done nothing together.

Rather than making up for teen's feelings of emotional deprivation in her relationship with mother, the arrival of step-Dad contributed to them:

> At first, when my mother married him, we um, you know, we wasn't getting along too good. He stopped talking to me. And I asked him to be friends, and we started being friends. I didn't want my Mom to remarry. I had wanted, you know, for her to stay single, separated, not, yea, single, cause when she wasn't married, you know, she spent a lot of time with us. She was around us all the time. When they married, she was still around, but you know, she had to like, give him attention too.

Mother B. This mother struggles hard to rationalize why her mother did not seem to love her. Although her mother virtually showered her with material things, she never said she loved her:

> I remember my Mama used to, used to give us anything we wanted. We had more candy than the average kids, you know. Anything we needed, we had everything. And, you know, I felt at one time that she didn't love me because I was the baby, but I seen, after she died, she was treating me that way because she knew I was supposed to be the best because my sister was an alcoholic, and my brother is an alcoholic, and they had been drinking ever since teenagers, you know, young teenagers. So, and I thought she didn't love me, but after she died, she left, her insurance policy was in my name, and I knew she was doing me that because she wanted me to be better than them. She knew I wasn't the type to drink and smoke. So, but I felt she didn't love me, but you know, she just didn't say she loved us. But I knew she was doing her best for us because we didn't go without anything. Like for special holidays we always would get the gifts we wanted. And birthdays, she didn't never forget them. Ummum, because like, you know, when special days would come, anything we said we wanted, she had it there for us. Like a new bike, rings, watches, anything we told her we wanted, she would get it for us. Just like when she would give me pretty dresses, just anything. She'd just go out her way to please us. From about, I can remember from about 5, 6, I used to wear dresses to school. Any time I said I wanted a new dress, she'd get me a dress. If she had the money, she'd get anything we said we needed or wanted, you know. Like when I used to go to the doctor, and she used to tell us "if you be good, I'll buy you a baby doll." And every time I'd

go to the doctor, she used to buy me a special treat. So now, when my kids go to the doctor and they be good, I'll go buy them a toy. That's what my Mama used to do us. And anything I said I wanted, she used to cook it. She used to bring my dinner to me, and I was a woman, you know. She still fix my dinner and bring it to me.

Mother struggles to justify her mother's beatings by blaming herself for them. But even this rationalization cannot explain why her mother never said she loved her:

She would holler at me, you know, she didn't have to hit me, cause that's the way my feelings was. And now, like I used to be in the house just mad, and she would, she beat me one time because I wasn't smiling. But after that, I seen it meant so much to her for me to be happy around her friends and her too. [How often did she beat you?] Maybe like twice, once or twice a month. It wasn't that much, but I hurt her when I be pouting and her friends used to come over. And I used to just stand up, looking out the door, mad and stuff, and I didn't even talk to her friends. She'd get mad and say I was ugly, you know, and I should respect them and talk to 'em. So when I changed my attitude like that then, you know, she started showing me that she cared, but she couldn't really say she loved me by having two alcoholics in the house, because they would feel she don't care about them, you know. And I guess she felt I could understand better. I told her I was tired of her wanting to hit on me when I wouldn't smile, and I was hurting inside. And then, that's when she started understanding how it feels. So, the doctor told her that if I don't want to smile, that's me. Leave me alone, you know. And that's when she stopped trying to make me smile.

Father abandoned his daughter before she was born. Even now, he sends mixed messages of love and rejection:

When I was conceived, my Daddy left before I was born. So um, I never wanted to meet him until I got older because I started having a problem, I couldn't deal with things cause I had so much inside of me I wanted to tell him. And so, one of my aunts that always, you know, his sister was saying I wasn't for him. So one of his other sisters, you know, she believed that I was his, so she fixed it so that he and I met. And from that day on, you know, when I feel I need to talk to him, I call him just to talk to him. But he don't call me, but I call him because I feel better when I talk to him. You know, after I told him how I felt toward him, I do feel better, just to talk to him every now and then. Yeah, he just left, and you know, he never came back. You know, my Mama never had heard from him until the welfare tracked him down because my Mama was on welfare. So like when Father's Day would come, I would send him a card because I had his address. And, you know, I wanted to reach out to him, but, you know, he just never wanted to admit that I was his. So, but now, you know, he, he feels, feels it now because like if he gets sick, and I call him, he say he be thinking about me and stuff like that.

This mother has insight that things might have turned out better if she had had a father or a mother to care for her and watch out for her:

Well, I know that it is very important to a child to have their father in their life, if they can, you know. Because I know how I feel now, you know. I get so depressed that if I just call my Daddy, it makes a big difference, you know. And when I tell him about things, sometimes he say "Take care of the kids, hear. I love you." You know, that's what he say sometimes, but sometimes he don't accept us. I think it, it affected me bad because I feel that if I would have had a father to discipline me, I would be a better person. I am not bad, because I don't do drugs and I don't smoke and I love my kids, and I want what's best for them, but if I would have had a Daddy in the house, I would be a whole, totally different person. Maybe I wouldn't have got pregnant without being married. And maybe I wouldn't have quit school, cause I quit school. See, 'cause my Mom used to go to work at like 6:30, and she didn't know whether I was going to school or not. But, you know, my sister did see to me, but if I'd tell 'em my stomach was hurting, I got to stay home. But I'm sorry that I quit school now. That's why I'm going back to finish it.

Her fear of talking to mother about important personal matters had fateful consequences:

[Discussing when she became pregnant for the first time] Just walked around, crying. I didn't have nobody to talk to. So, I just kept everything in. She never did say anything because, you see, she'd be working. I was scared to tell my Mama. My sister was the one that told me (about sex). Because you see, my Mama never told us about, you know, don't, all she would say was keep your dress down, you know. But she never did say why. Because like she did tell us "Don't take money from men," O.K. So when I started going out with my oldest Daddy, he used to want to give me money, I just said "No, I don't want it." He used to say "You're the first woman I see that don't want money." But she really didn't explain it to me, you know, like if you're going out with a guy, you can take it [the money] but, I was pregnant, and didn't want to take money from him until I realized I was wrong. She didn't mean it like that. She meant, you know, to not have sex with him.

Competitive

Teen. The themes of being "Daddy's girl," of having an alliance with Daddy that excludes mother, and of Daddy protecting daughter from mother's hostility are illustrated in this teen's interview. Mother is portrayed as mean, lacking in understanding, depriving, and rejecting, whereas father is portrayed as the opposite of those characteristics.

I would creep by my Daddy, anything I did I would run to my Daddy. Sometimes I couldn't tell my Mama things, but I always could tell my Daddy everything! Like when I got hit by a car when I was little. He was, I didn't want my Mama to touch me. 'Cause I thought she was gonna be mad and be mean, but my Daddy was right there, he helped me get quiet and stuff, he was right there. I was scared, and I didn't want to go by nobody but Daddy, and he was still, I feel closer to my Daddy because I can tell him about anything. Like, when I came up pregnant, I couldn't tell my Mama, but I could tell my Daddy. You know, to me he's more understanding. He gets things done the right way. Maybe because when you talk with her about something, she fusses a lot. You know, you didn't want to hear all that fussing, you just wanted to talk to her. But she get upset and start fussing and stuff.

The fussing that teen and her sisters did not want to hear about had to do with their adolescent sexuality:

She used to tell us that we don't need no baby, that we need education more and she said we didn't, we don't know how to really cope with no children because we was children ourselves. And then, you know, we used to talk in the hall, "Mama we don't want to hear that" and stuff like that. And she used to be good and mad, but we would used to leave, go where we wouldn't hear it.

Mother's rage and father's role as confidant and protector came into sharp focus when teen became pregnant:

[When Teen's mother found out she was pregnant] Well she did-n't, she was mad but she didn't say nothing because my Daddy knew how she was going to react, so he told her not to tell me nothing. He talked to me about the responsibilities and things. And he talked to the baby's Daddy, and everything was taken care of through my Daddy because my Mama, she was upset and mad and stuff. She told me she had drew the last straw with me. She didn't mean it.

If teen felt deprived by mother before her pregnancy, she feels more so now that baby is born:

Well, it's okay, but you know you have to take on so many responsibilities, and you get less now than you used to. Like my Mom used to give me money every weekend, she don't do that now. She, you know, she give me money but not like she used to. Because, maybe, because I already be having it and it's like you have to watch out, you got someone else to watch out for more than yourself. And you just have to buy things for someone more than yourself. You just get less than you used to.

Mother. In this interview, the mother of childhood—a woman prone to chastising daughter when Daddy was not home to protect her—is con-trasted with the mother of adulthood—a woman whose nurturance and participation in rearing her grandchildren were greatly desired by this mother. Her special relationship with father in childhood and adulthood, and later her relationship with her own man, have come between mother and herself, to her great regret and sorrow. This mother's love for her mother and yearning for a close relationship with mother as an adult are especially poignant.

This mother was special in her family and in the affections of her father until the birth of another girl 9 years later, an event to which she did not take kindly:

I was just like [her own daughter's name]. I was a "Daddy's girl." I was the only girl for 9 years. And when my sister next to me was born, she was a pretty, pretty baby, and looked like they used to give her all the attention you know. And my Mama told me one day for me to watch her. I told her I wasn't watching no baby, 'cause I didn't have no babies. And I was upstairs playing, 'cause we used to keep all our toys up there. And uh, I had a dog, and she just attacked the dog. And I pushed her down the stairs, cause I didn't want no sister. Them boys was all right, but I didn't want no sisters.

She could get away with acts of revenge against siblings as long as Daddy was home, but when he was not, she was in trouble:

And like the boys used to come and play with my brothers, and if they didn't want me to play, I'd set 'em on fire. You know, like on Fridays, they used to cut the grass, and they didn't want me to get up under the house and play with them, and I'd get some newspaper and stick it under the grass and make it smoke, and after I'd run and jump on my Daddy's lap, and act like I didn't be who did that. Yeah, my Daddy didn't allow me to catch whuppings. But when my Daddy wasn't home, Mama used to whup me with anything, pots, pans.

She could count on her Daddy to fuss at mother for "whupping" her:

When I was young, I used to do anything to get off with him. I remember one time my Mama told me to wash dishes and I didn't wash them. And she would whip me. And I was standing on the front porch, and I seen my Daddy coming home. And I run to the corner and I met him, and I told him. And him and my Mama started fussing.

But when she got older, Daddy disappointed and rejected her:

And then he got that, he started running around with this woman. I didn't even know my Daddy was running around. All I know is he left when I was 15, and that was it. And he never came back since. And then he said I wasn't his. He said I was for somebody else. And even right up until today, I think about that, 'cause I remembered it.

When Daddy got sick, he and daughter renewed their special relationship:

I remember, even when he got down to sleep, he used to just cry, cry, cry. 'Cause he came home to go to sleep, but he'd want to sleep with my Mama, and my Mama told him, No, he couldn't sleep with her, 'cause he had left her when she was sick. So he called me, like, he made me come out. I told him, yeah, he could come stay with me. But that was his idea, it wasn't none of mine. And he used to just cry, cry, cry. And I used to always ask him what he was crying for, and he'd say I was always his favorite, "even as bad I used to be," he would say, "You the only one who takes me." He said, "I had to come back to you." I said, "Well, this is your house," I say, "It ain't mine, you know, but I done it for you." And me and him growed close, 'til that, you know, it was that time.

As an adult and mother of her own children, this mother yearned for her mother's love, care, attention, and help in raising her children, but she received these things only sparingly because she had a man in the house.

And like when I had my first child, my Mama used to be with me. And uh, like I would be sick, you know, and she used to come help us. She would have moods though. "How you have to . . ." she said. You know, me and the children's Daddy, we weren't married, we were just staying together. And she told me she was going, cause she knowed I had a good man. And she left then, and like I used to ask the Lord, you know, for to take me, before he would take my Mama, you know, because I couldn't stand it, you know. Well, there was my Mama, gone just like she had died. And she was supposed to be coming back, and she didn't come back. She stayed, and I used to call every day, and she used to tell me she was coming, and then she started saying the childrens didn't want her to come home. And when I was pregnant with the oldest girl, she didn't come home at all.

She substituted mother's blouse for mother when mother left again:

But I was sick with the youngest girl, 'cause she was a breech, and then she came home. That's when she stayed, for 6 months, she helped me with her. And after she left, I started having trouble with the baby, cause she didn't want to sleep at night. So I had, I own a blouse my Mama had back then, and I used to wrap the baby in that blouse. After I just be doing it, I used to couldn't even wash it.

Mature

Teen. In this family, grandmother took care of teen while mother worked. Grandmother was the disciplinarian, and mother was the parent figure who encouraged teen's growth and development. All three women in the family are represented in this interview as mutually involved in promoting separation and individuation within themselves and each other in the context of relationships based on emotional understanding and mutual respect. As teen describes, however, movement toward increasing autonomy for teen generated anxieties and conflicts for all three women.

> Grandmother raised me a bit more than Mom, but Mom was always there for me. When the other kids teased me in kindergarten, she said "Your real friend is your Mother, don't worry about it if the other kids tease you because I'll always love you." She was patient in teaching me when she didn't want to do it. She paid attention to my homework even though she was tired after work. She helped me learn to ride a bike with training wheels even when I was ready to give up until finally I learned. She gave me advice about cooking, and anything I needed help with. She gave me a computer. . . . She's loving, she takes me to visit friends when I'm lonely in the summer. . . . Both took care of me when I was sick, and held me a lot.

Teen's perspective is that grandmother is behind the times with regards to what teenagers are doing these days, and she resents mother's agreement with grandmother about these matters. However, teen understands their anxieties and concerns and takes an educational rather than an oppositional approach to the problem:

> My grandmother was stricter, she had an earlier curfew, and my mother always goes along with her. I resent that sometimes. . . . My Mom and my Grandmom treated me like I was younger when I became a teen—they wouldn't let me go to a party if they didn't know the person giving it too well. I just started using examples that all my friends were going to be there and I'd be back home early. It's hard for Mom and Grandmother to understand how things are now for teens. They were raised differently. Like the prom, they didn't go out to eat before a prom or have parties after. Both are sort of surprised, but they understand and they are getting better with all these, they just want to raise me the way they was raised. . . . They would discipline me for showing disrespect.

It got worse in the first part of my teen years, but it's improved, and I see it going back to like it was in childhood.

Just as teen helps mother and grandmother to loosen their ties to her, grandmother helps teen to do the same:

I was separated from them when I went to Upward Bound over the summer. I called home every day until my grandmother told me I was running the phone bill up.

Teen acknowledges feeling rejected in the past that mother chose to work instead of spending time with her. At this point in her development, however, teen identifies with mother's and grandmother's own self-sufficiency, self-discipline, and ability to love, as well as with their aspirations for her in these regards:

I felt rejected because Mom wouldn't take family vacations, but I realized she didn't have time. I worried about Mom staying out late at work but Mom explained she was just doing it to help me, so we could live better. . . . My experiences with Mom and Grandmother taught me how to love, how to earn things instead of just wanting somebody to give it to you. And how to discipline myself. And work. I guess they tried to make me feel more confident about myself.

At the same time that teen aspires to be independent, she recognizes the pull toward remaining dependent on mother and grandmother—a pull she feels she must resist:

I have plans to go to Howard. I think I really need to get by myself for once, 'cause I never really been that far away from home. And I need to learn how to be more independent, 'cause I've become dependent on my mother and grandmother too much. I would wish for my mother and grandmother to always be together forever, and to be happy and getting along with my mother and grandmother, and to have a big family. My most significant experience I guess would be leaving home and being by myself for the first time this summer. I realized how much I would miss my mother and grandmother, and how to be by myself.

Mother. The predominant theme in this interview is of mother identifying with her own mother's strength of character, kindness, and ability to survive under austere economic conditions:

Around holidays we were very happy. She like to bake cakes, and she would make huge, good towering cakes, you know, real, real good cakes. They were delicious. She just made everybody feel welcome and we had no money but whatever she could, we just had a lot. She'd stretch regardless of what you had so she could clean it, if it was a rag, wash that rag and let it be the cleanest rag you had. Your socks, you had one pair, so you wash that pair, put it on tomorrow. Nobody knows what pair it was. Mom taught the value of money, economize, you know, not wasting. You don't have very much money, and just because you have a dime and just because you see something, if you don't need it, think about it twice and don't just go spend that dime because you have it and you never had a dime before, think about where you going to place it, if it's of value.

Being the youngest in the family gave her more opportunities to be with her mother and to learn from her:

I was the youngest, always under her, I lived with her until she died. Out in the garden, she would plant corn or string beans or what have you, okra, a vegetable garden. And I would always be under her, around her, so she and I would always be talking. And I would enjoy it. I'm the youngest.

Although her mother disciplined her with whippings and did not hold her much, this mother did not feel rejected because these were the customs in those days:

My Mom's mother died when Mom was young, so she had to grow up in a hurry, so she experienced a lot, and just had patience. She gave us whuppings if we didn't obey. She didn't have to do it often because you would recall what she did the other time. I guess you call whupping abuse, and nowadays, that may be true, don't you think? I wasn't held much by Mom—parents at that time didn't hug and do all that to children. But still and all, nobody had all of that, so you didn't feel rejected. I sort of like the way I was reared, children then . . . but I mean it won't work now, but I like it you know.

This mother is clear about her identification with her mother's strengths and aspirations for daughter's progressive development toward maturity; self-sufficiency; and an intimate, stable relationship with a man of her own:

I'm very much like her. I try to make those cakes, and cook, but I'm not as good (at cooking) as she was. I think I'm sort of kind, she was a kind person. I try to listen and find out what she says, cause I spent a lot of time with my mother. She got more concerned about my whereabouts when I got my period at age 10, and told me to "keep that dress down." In that time, according to the things my mother taught us, girls didn't have babies that did not marry. In my teen years, our relationship looked more mature like. Mom wanted me to go out and have dates and find someone really nice to marry. She wanted the best for me.

Mother's way of relating internally with her own mother is carried over in the representation of her relationship with her own daughter. Mother expresses satisfaction about daughter's identifications with her and tolerance of the ways in which daughter wants to be different:

This is the first year she's beginning to branch out and listen to loud music. She does think a little, wholeheartedly, just the way I think about things, because she believes in each individual person, you know, thinks about the whole self-concept, and I have nothing to say against that. I think it's good. Because she believes that the total, there are certain things that make up the total person, and I think that's fine. I'm learning from her, you understand, because there's more to an individual than one side. So I feel like she feels that, I know she thinks when she's not around me she acts like I act, do certain things I do. "Mama, I fix that just like you fix it," you know, like if it's some food. "I can fix that just like you weren't there and I fix that just like you, and more and more I find I just seeing certain things just like you." I said good [spoken very softly].

Mother. This mother represents her own mother as loving and firm but sometimes able to understand and respect daughter's individuality. In mother's relationship with her own daughter, she identifies with many of her mother's qualities:

Well, it was sometimes smooth and rough. Um, she was understanding at times and other times she wasn't. We were emotional. We could sit down as mother and daughter and talk about different situations that we encountered as far as myself and growing up and she had a way to make things right. You know, if I had a situation that I couldn't handle she would sit me down and we'd talk about it, explain to me, you know, the facts of life if

you want to call it that. And at the end of the conversation everything was fine. Like having a rough time with the fellas at school,
guys, peer pressure, you know, like dealing with them at an adolescent stage into a more adult stage and then trying to cope with
saying "yes" and "no" and then she'd bring out the Bible and
we'd go from there. She taught me morals how to be a lady and
respect myself, that kind of thing.

At times I felt that I was totally right in decision making. She
would be right there firm you know, with a firm grip saying "No
you are not right." Like wanting to move away from home at the
age of 16 and I hadn't completed my high school yet and the reason for that like I said we ran away from hurricanes a lot. And
after the hurricane was over we could move back home and
because she was not going to move back, you know. I was just
ready to move out and she as firm and said "No, you will not.
You will finish school and you will stay here." You know. It
worked out.

My mom was a pretty hard woman to deal with you know as far
as getting her to change her mind. Going out to parties. If I
wanted to go out to a party and I would practically beg her and
it was hard for me but you know I understand now because I
have a daughter and when she wants to just go and I can't find
any sense into her going she doesn't go. I think that was the main
thing to just go ahead on and keep me away from a lot of things
that would disturb our life style. She's still like that today. She's
still rough, still rough. She's hard to change her mind, but once
she changes her mind you know that's when the understanding
comes in. And that when I can finally understand. Like understanding she [her daughter] wanted to play softball instead of bas-
ketball, participate in band instruments, involved in little
sweetheart things. I guess that's a part of understanding.

Mother identifies with her own mother's valuing of relationships with
men, despite the many problems and difficulties associated with these
relationships:

When I went through my first marriage and it was rough in my
marriage and I couldn't figure out how she managed. You know,
she lived with my father all those years before she left him and I
was ready to leave my husband when I married him 2 weeks after
I married him. She said "Hang in there, you can do it." Finally
after 7 years I divorced. I stopped listening to her, and it took her
a while to deal with it and then she had to understand, she

accepted it and my new husband. It took her a while. That's the rough side. But she went through a divorce and how difficult it is to train the children with new stepfathers and mothers and she pretty much didn't want my daughter to go through that.

The combined emotionalities of mother and daughter sometimes led to ruptures in their relationship, but none that could not be repaired and coped with by two mature adults:

She loves children, she said "I wish I had of kept that child" [mother's daughter]. She takes in everybody, her home is open to everybody, she's that kind of person. She was not overprotective, she was very protective of her children. She gets emotional when the kids disobey, like when I took candy out of one of my brother's Easter baskets, and when I spent my lunch money when she said not to. And then I turned out emotionally upset with her one day and wouldn't let her touch me anymore. That was when I thought I was grown. Even now we still get upset at each other once in a while but we're able to cope because we're both adults.

Her mother's aspirations for her emanated from a position of empathy:

I'm closer to Mom because she was there most of the time. All the time, and she said she made me look at my life and really want to know exactly what I could get as far as gold stars. She didn't pressure me into being something that I knew I couldn't be but she tried to, you know, she instilled enough, you know, in my head to where I could want to do what I could and not try to downgrade myself or anything but always keep my head up. That kind of thing, be somebody.

Her mother and father were both valued parents, but for different qualities and functions:

He [Dad] was the breadwinner, she was the disciplinarian, she was the educator, she was there for whatever. She was the voice when we needed the voice to tell us how to go about doing things. She was the one to put us to bed, get us up. She was just there, you know. She didn't really work any place but she was a home-maker. She made me do housework, laundry, showed me the ropes. And in spite of all the things that I thought she was doing wrong, I find myself teaching my daughter, you have to do these things. You have to know how to manage. You have to get out on your own one day. You know, that's the kind of things she would tell me.

(Father) wasn't home a lot because of his work. He really didn't get into the family too much. If I needed him to do something, he did it without any questions usually or he would be easy in his ways. I could talk him into anything. He would be right there to take me, you know, if he were at home. I think basically that's what it was because he worked so much. We understood that he wasn't home all the time. When we needed him there he wasn't there but when he was there he would be do what he could. And he wasn't the disciplinarian type. He loved his kids and would do what he can when he was there. Whatever it took, he was a good provider. He was a very good provider. He didn't get too emotional. He was just jolly old Dad. Even today, he's still jolly old Dad. I loved him and even today I still don't see him as often. He don't stay home a lot. And when we do get together he tries to make as much as he can out that little time that we spend but that's the only closeness, physical closeness I know. The mental things are there and you know I have a deep desire there where I wish all of my family could be as close as they could possibly be.

Sometimes her mother relied on father for the disciplining:

He would give me a talk for about 15 or 20 minutes, you know and in between I would have to answer some questions and when I'd go to babbling and crying, he would say "Well now, you know, Daddy has to talk to you and tell you these things because I'm only doing it because I want you to do what's right." And I would just be bawling and say "Can I go blow my nose." That's what he did, you know. It helped. He did spank us when we took the watermelon. My Mama said "It's outta my hands, I don't want to do it." She said "You take care of 'em," and he knew she wanted us to get a spanking then. So he went ahead on and spanked us. That's the only time I can remember my Dad spanking.

Her mother and father were not perfect, but they set the stage for her development:

It's a learning space being a parent, being a husband and a wife. First, you know, learning to be married then learning to be a parent and then having children to raise and it's a lifetime thing. They were pretty good parents overall. I have no regrets as far as them being parents and how they acted and reacted to situations. I think they did pretty well. They set the stage for us.

PROPERTIES OF INTERNAL WORKING MODELS

Quality of Thought

One dimension of individual differences in adolescents' and adults' representations of attachment relationships identified in this chapter pertains to quality of thought, or what others in the attachment literature have termed *states of mind* (Main, 1995) or *internal working models* (Bretherton, 1985). This construct is conceived here as how respondents say what they say on the AAI and refers to such characteristics as quantity of verbal output and the capacity or willingness to retrieve past feelings and thoughts related to attachment experiences, to integrate seemingly contradictory feelings and thoughts, to reflect insightfully on remembered attachment-related experiences, to recognize and acknowledge the importance of attachment-related events, and to allow oneself to feel and to express feelings about attachment experiences and figures in the interview situation.

The descriptive properties of quality-of-thought categories emerging from our qualitative analyses of AAIs with adolescent girls and their mothers were quite similar to properties identified by Main, Kobak, and other attachment researchers for secure, preoccupied, and dismissing internal working model categories—hence, we adopted the same category labels. The quality-of-thought classifications we assigned to individuals in this study using qualitative methods corresponded closely to the classifications we assigned on the basis of quantitative multivariate analyses of Q-sort item scores. Further, the latter classifications were highly correlated with those derived using Kobak's prototype correlation method.[1]

These similarities and correlations do not mean that our quality-of-thought constructs in this and in attachment research are equivalent or interchangeable or that the findings from this study can be directly compared to findings from studies using the quality-of-thought (state of mind, internal working model) construct as operationally defined by Main's coding system. These similarities and correlations do suggest, however, that our quality-of-thought construct is measuring something at least remotely related to the construct measured by Main's coding scheme for the AAI

---

[1] Chapter 4, Table 4-1.

and by Kobak's Adult Attachment Q-sort. The issue of the relation between the quality-of-thought construct in this research and Main's (1995) conceptualization of adults' states of mind about attachment is addressed in greater depth in the final section of chapter 7.

Analyses further indicated that quality-of-thought and the thematic content–structure dimensions are separate, although perhaps related, components of internal working models, thus justifying our use of separate quality-of-thought and "working model proper" measures.[2] In so doing, we are able later in this chapter to empirically examine in the context of our sample an important but untested assumption of attachment theory—that preoccupied and dismissing qualities of thought are associated with unfavorable attachment-related experiences, whereas the secure quality is associated with either favorable or unfavorable experiences (e.g., Kobak & Sceery, 1988; Main, 1995; Main et al., 1985).

Measuring quality of thought and thematic content separately also allows for a more precise understanding of other issues and relations of interest to us and to attachment researchers. These include intergenerational concordances in attachment representations, relations between mothers' working models of their own and their daughters' attachment relationships, and relations between working models and sociocultural and behavioral variables including family environments, cultural schemas, and adolescent pregnancy outcomes. In previous attachment research, for example, intergenerational concordances have been found between classifications of parents and their children on the AAI (e.g., Benoit, Vidovic, & Roman, 1991) and between parents' classifications on the AAI and their infants' classifications on the Strange Situation (Benoit et al., 1991; Crowell & Feldman, 1988; Fonagy et al., 1991). Because determination of classifications on the AAI in these studies has relied on a measure combining quality of thought and what we have termed working model proper criteria, it is not clear whether concordances in these other studies reflect intergenerational continuity in quality of thought, working models proper (content), or both. Separating out the two components of the internal working model variable allows for a more direct assessment in our sample of this and similar questions.

Internal Working Models Proper

The second dimension of individual differences in working models identified in this study consists of the predominant themes and levels of structural differentiation and integration reflected in respondents' representations of attachment relationships, or internal working models proper. Conceptually,

---

[2] Appendix A, part B-1.

themes and levels of structural differentiation and integration are two sides of the same coin. Both are revealed by what respondents say with regard to their representations of attachment relationships. From this perspective, internal working models proper could be thought of as what respondents are talking about rather than how they are talking about it. They reflect a mixture of conscious and unconscious memories, wishes, beliefs, and affects pertaining to respondents' relationships with attachment figures that are tied together or integrated in a storyline that has both content and structure.

Structural properties of models pertain, for example, to the degree to which boundaries between self and other are represented as blurred or maintained; the degree to which roles belonging to self, mother, and father are confused, homogenized, or differentiated; whether relationships represented are primarily dyadic, triadic, or more complex; or the degree to which childhood attachment figures (mother and father figures) remain or have been replaced as primary sources and objects of instinctual/affective investment.

Themes reflect respondents' often-conflicting goals and desires vis-à-vis attachment figures, their thoughts, and feelings about themselves and others as they engage in the process of relating; their characteristic modes of attempting to satisfy wants or express feelings; their expectations and anticipations regarding the consequences of such attempts; and the defensive methods by which respondents protect themselves from anticipated dangers and anxiety. The ways that women in this study described their mental and behavioral interactions with attachment figures are clearly reminiscent of the descriptions given by Erik Erikson (1963) of characteristic ways that infants, toddlers, and young children relate intrapsychicaly and interpersonally to others. This correspondence is important because Erikson's descriptions are grounded in a theory that can provide at least a beginning framework for understanding where internal working models proper come from and what forces are at work in shaping individual pathways of development.

Structurally less differentiated and integrated deprived models of adolescents and adults emphasize themes reminiscent of Erikson's (1963) descriptions of the first two phases of infantile psychosexual and ego development.[3] These are themes of wanting to get what has not been given freely, wanting to take and hold onto emotional and material supplies, and wanting to give and give up valuable possessions and aspects

---

[3] Erikson named these phases or periods in the child's development according to the bodily zones and functions that ascend in importance relative to others at a given time or according to the ego qualities that emerge from conflicts characteristic of a given phase. Thus, the earliest childhood developmental phase is named mouth and senses, or basic trust versus mistrust; the second is named eliminative organs and musculature, or autonomy versus shame and doubt; the third is named locomotion and the genitals, or initiative versus guilt.

of the self to others, together with the associated pleasures, disappoint-ments, frustrations, struggles, and battles that ensue in the process of attempting to satisfy these wants. Throughout these interviews are clear themes of yearning to be close, to trust, to be cared for, and to care for others, offset by a wish to be in control, to resist control of others, to rebell, to be separate and autonomous, and to protect oneself from the anticipated dangers of closeness. In deprived models, these themes are expressed in the context of dyadic relationships.

More differentiated competitive models separate out self from other, mother from father, and integrate these distinct person representations in complex and multifaceted relationships. Themes in the competitive model described in this study emphasize competition with mother for the affec-tions of father, together with the desire to atone for these competitive wishes and to maintain the love and affections of mother. When the little girl desires a special place in father's affections—that is, to be Daddy's girl—mother is represented simultaneously as an enemy to be displaced or otherwise neutralized by father's interventions and a figure from whom the little girl continues to desire nurturance, caring, and love. Thus, although competitive respondents desire access to both parents, they attempt to gain access not only to elicit a sensitive, empathic response or protection and comfort from a parent, but also to play the role of confi-dant or spouse vis-à-vis father, combined with the complementary one of blocking access by a mother perceived as threatening or intruding. These goals presuppose a triadic representational structure and emphasize the social modality of "being on the make," a phrase suggesting "head-on attack, enjoyment of competition, insistence on goal, pleasure of con-quest" (Erikson, 1963, p. 255).

Daughters with mature working models proper represent themselves as identifying with mothers' values, interests, and talents; mothers' ways of thinking and coping with life's challenges; ways of relating with men; and aspirations for daughters' capacities to become independent, to be autonomous, and to have a family of their own. Rather than competing with mother for the attentions and affections of father (or stepfathers, grandmothers, boyfriends, etc.), mature daughters accept and value moth-ers' other attachment relationships and strive to become like mother in forming new attachment relationships of their own. Through these iden-tifications, daughters describe themselves as becoming more and more like mother at the same time that they are becoming more and more emanci-pated from her and other primary attachment ties (e.g., father, stepfather, grandmother). Put in structural terms, mature models reflect both a fur-ther differentiation and a further integration in daughters' representations of attachment relationships. Put in thematic terms, goals of mature respon-dents emphasize the social modalities of winning recognition, producing, and achieving, becoming one's own competent person through the internalization (internal reconstruction) of the admired competencies, characteristics, and attributes of parents. The mature respondent in this study fits Erikson's (1963) description of the child who has moved into the phase of industry versus inferiority. She has "experienced a sense of finality regarding the fact that there is no workable future within the womb of the family, and thus becomes ready to apply [her]self to given skills and tasks which go far beyond the mere playful expression of the organ modes or the pleasure in the function of [her] limbs" (p. 259).

In all three models, representations of mothers cannot be adequately understood outside of the context of father representations, and vice versa. In deprived working models, for example, the highly ambivalent and relatively undifferentiated "deprived" representation of the mother–daughter relationship is paralleled and is partly explained by a concomitant representation of father as depriving. The representation in the competitive working model of mother as a hostile intruder in daughter's hoped-for exclusive relationship with father is understandable only in the context of daughter's representation of self as Daddy's girl and of father as sweet, affectionate, understanding, and ready to come to her rescue in the face of mother's unreasonable demands and behavior. The representation in the mature working model of mother as a woman to be emulated, identified with, and yet emancipated from has as a background a representation of father and men in general as potentially capable of serving useful and welcomed functions in the lives of both mother and daughter, regardless of whether these functions are currently or have ever been served by actual fathers.

In terms of both structure and thematic content, then, deprived, competitive, and mature working models proper can be arranged in that order along a continuum from least to most "developed" and are best understood from a developmental perspective. Unanswered questions about working models proper arising from a developmental point of view include the following: What are the processes whereby internal working models proper develop? What accounts for individual variations among models? What does it mean that an adolescent or adult would retain characteristics of an earlier childhood mode of thinking and relating in her current representations of attachment relationships? What are the interactions between quality of thought and working models proper in development? To find answers to these questions, a theoretical framework is needed that can not only accommodate the descriptive properties of internal working models proper in the fullness of their being, but offers a logically coherent, internally consistent, and comprehensive explanation of how models come into being.

Erikson's Theory of Development

Erikson's (1963) theoretical framework goes part of the way toward accomplishing these goals. His theory emphasizes the interactions and interrelations among instinctual/affective forces within the individual, on the one hand, and forces coming from the "maternal environment," on the other hand, in the ultimate shaping and molding of psychic representations and individual proclivities toward social modalities. In this focus, Erikson's views fit well with those of Hans Loewald (1980), whose theoretical framework I believe is well-suited to accommodate the internal working models proper construct and whose ideas I describe in greater detail in the next chapter.

In Erikson's (1963) view, dominant social modes of relating and their affective concomitants are evident in the behavioral and psychic productions of individuals of all ages. These dominant modes of relating, moreover, are "anchored in the groundplan of the body" (p. 108). At successive phases of physical maturation, different bodily zones assume dominance in the intrapsychic and interpersonal life of the child. These zones are, in temporal order of ascendance, the "mouth and senses," "the elimination and musculature zones," and the "locomotor and genital" zones. That certain bodily zones ascend in importance at a given phase does not mean for Erikson that those associated with previous phases fade out or away, but rather that zones that had been relatively less important in earlier phases assume relatively more importance for the child, partly because of maturational development and partly because of the expectations of the maternal environment, a term that for Erikson subsumes an ever-widening circle of realms in the child's interpersonal world.

The significance of bodily zones in the intrapsychic world of the child, said Erikson (1963), is that each has its own characteristic mode of functioning. The mouth and senses systems function to incorporate, to get, to take in, and to more actively go after things to bite on, through, and off things (pp. 75–77). The eliminative organs and musculature zones function to retain and eliminate, to flex and extend, and to relax and maintain rigidity. The locomotor and genitals systems function to intrude, to include, to thrust, and to ambulate. Erikson said,

> the mode of intrusion is suggested in ambulatory exuberance, in aggressive mentality, in sexual fantasies and activities. Both sexes partake of the general development of ambulatory and intrusive patterns, although in the girl patterns of demanding and mothering inception develop in a ratio determined by previous experience, temperament and cultural emphasis. (p. 88)

Organ functions, however, do not translate directly into modes of relating to others intrapsychically or interpersonally. Social modalities in Erikson's view are not automatic, inevitable by-products of maturation in organ systems, as some interpreters of Erikson would suggest. Representations may be anchored in the groundwork of the body, but in no way are these representations simple readouts of a biological maturational sequence. Rather, the infant or child has to learn to use her organ systems in ways that accord both with what she is equipped to do best and with the expectations and patterns of the maternal environment.

Erikson (1963) said that two things can interfere with this learning. One is a loss of inner control. A second is a breakdown in the mutuality between child and caregiver. For a newborn, for example, the most general mode of approach toward the external world and mother is that of receptive incorporation, manifested by the "taking in" of "materia" through the mouth, eyes, ears, and skin and through attempts to grasp. However, alongside this mode that dominates the newborn stage there is also a "clamping down with jaws and gums" (the active incorporative mode), a "spitting up and out" (the eliminative mode), "the closing up of the lips" (the retentive mode), and even a "general intrusive tendency of the whole head and neck . . . to fasten itself upon the nipple, and as it were, into the breast" (p. 73). A disturbance of either inner control or mutual regulation may bring what is ordinarily an auxiliary mode into "near dominance" (p. 73).

To continue the example, an infant with pyloric spasm, which thrusts food out again shortly after intake, routinely experiences the eliminative mode with what is usually the dominant receptive incorporative mode. A consequence may be an overdevelopment of the retentive mode, an oral closing up, which "becomes a generalized mistrust of whatever comes in because it is apt not to stay" (p. 75). Similarly, a mother's habitual withdrawal of the breast "because she has been nipped or fears she will be" may prompt the infant to prematurely develop the biting reflex. This situation, said Erikson, can be a model for a radical disturbance in interpersonal relations. As he put it, "one hopes to get, the source is withdrawn, whereupon one tries reflexively to hold onto and to take; but the more one holds on, the more determinedly does the source remove itself" (p. 75).

What is most important for development in Erikson's (1963) view, then, is the mutuality between what the infant is predisposed to do as a matter of course and what the mother wants or expects for the infant. "Whatever reaction patterns are given biologically and whatever schedule is predetermined developmentally must be considered to be a series of potentialities for changing patterns of mutual regulation" (p. 75). The expectable sequence is one that will play out if the child is able to regulate his or her organ systems "in accordance with the way in which the maternal environment integrates its methods of child care" (p. 75).

Internal working models proper, in the context of Erikson's ideas, reflect an individual's dominant mode of thinking and relating internally to attachment figures and attachment-related events. This dominant mode is the present realization of a potential for relating in particular ways, which has come about through the conjoint participation of child and the maternal environment, or through the mutual regulation of what is expected and what is given or develops naturally or unnaturally. This dominant mode is of the present, is related to the past in a way that cannot be determined without additional knowledge of an individual's intrapsychic history, and is not necessarily determinative of the future. Patterns of mutual regulation between an individual and the social environment may change, as may the internal representations of these patterns.

RELATIONS AMONG AND BETWEEN MOTHERS' AND DAUGHTERS' PERSONAL REPRESENTATIONS

Cohort Differences

As we did for family environment, cultural schema, and adolescent pregnancy variables in chapter 5, we now address questions of how respondents' mental representations of attachment relationships fit together with each other and with adolescent pregnancy. The first question asked has to do with generational trends; in particular, how do older mothers, younger mothers, and teen cohorts in this sample differ with respect to classifications on the internal working model proper and quality-of-thought variables? Comparisons of frequencies of older mothers, younger mothers, and teens in the three main internal working model proper categories revealed a trend toward greater numbers of older mothers in the competitive category and fewer numbers of older mothers in the deprived category relative to younger mothers and teens. Percentages of mature mothers did not differ across cohorts.[4] No reliable cohort differences were observed for the quality-of-thought variable.

Relations Among Personal Representational Variables and Adolescent Pregnancy

In this section, our focus is on relations among the various kinds of personal representations and with adolescent pregnancy, both within and

---

[4] Percentages of older mothers, younger mothers, and teens in the deprived category were 11, 35, and 30; in the competitive category were 55, 39, and 35; and in the mature

between cohorts. Figure 1 summarizes findings from loglinear analyses in graphic form. A summary of these findings in plain English are presented in the following paragraphs. Specific details of the analyses are presented in footnotes and in Appendix D.[5]

Overview of findings. In both cohorts, women's internal working models proper—that is, their intrapsychic representations of themselves in relationships with parental attachment figures—strongly predicted whether they had become adolescent mothers or had delayed pregnancy until they were older and married. In contrast, the quality of thought that women exhibited when discussing these relationships in interviews, although related in both cohorts to the structural and content components of working models (working models proper), did not predict adolescent pregnancy outcomes in either cohort.[6]

Mothers' beliefs that daughters preferred mothers over fathers, fathers over mothers, or valued both parental relationships equally (labeled Mom's Rep of Teen in Figure 1) were less closely associated with daughters' own representations of these relationships (Teen's IWM-p) than with mothers' representations of their own childhood attachment relationships (Mom's IWM-p). Mom's Rep of Teen and Teen's IWM-p had compounding, multiplicative effects on the odds of daughters' adolescent pregnancy outcomes.

Adolescent pregnancy outcomes as a function of representational variables. Teens' IWM-p were strong predictors of their adolescent pregnancy status. The same basic finding held true for mothers of these adolescent girls. In both cohorts, deprived women were highly likely to have been pregnant as adolescents, competitive women were slightly more likely to have become pregnant as teenagers than not, and mature women were unlikely to have been pregnant as adolescents.[7]

category were 34, 27, and 36. Chi-square tests revealed significant differences in internal working model proper classifications between older and younger mothers, $\chi^2(2, N = 87) = 6.87, p < .05$; and between older mothers and teens, $\chi^2(2, N = 125) = 6.94, p < .05$.

[5] A series of loglinear analyses was performed to examine relations among mothers' or teens' adolescent pregnancy outcomes and the representational variables constructed in this chapter. Each analysis in the series conformed to the general description of loglinear analyses presented in Appendix C (C-1) and discussed in chapter 5. In order to maximize the ratio of participants to cells, only three variables were included in each analysis.

[6] These findings pertain to the quality-of-thought construct as derived through our methods and therefore may or may not reflect what might be found with regard to quality of thought as constructed through Main's or Kobak's coding procedures. Both Main and Kobak's quality-of-thought constructs, as previously discussed, include descriptors of what people say about their attachment relationships and *how* they say it. Our construct, in contrast, focuses exclusively on *how* people talk about their relationships, with the content of interviews providing the basis for a separate construct (internal working models proper).

[7] The first two analyses in the series looked at relations among the internal working

Figure 6-1. Associations Among Adolescent Pregnancy and
Representational Variables

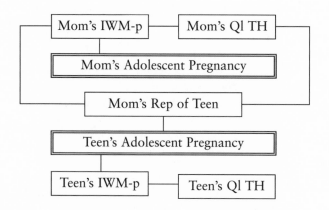

Although the relationship was not as strong when looked at from the other direction, pregnant women in both cohorts were more likely to remember their childhood attachment relationships through deprived or competitive than mature lenses, and never-pregnant women were more likely to remember these relationships in accordance with mature models.

Mom's Rep of Teen also made a difference with regard to daughters' pregnancy outcomes. Regardless of Teens' IWM-p, mothers who resentfully depicted daughters as Daddy's girl [Bad Mom (BM)/Good Dad(GD)] most likely to have pregnant daughters, followed by mothers who represented daughters' relationships with themselves as relatively better than with fathers [Mixed Mom (MM)/Bad Dad (BD)], followed by mothers who depicted both parental relationships positively [Good Mom (GM)/Good Dad(GD)].[8] It can be seen from the numbers in Table 6-4 that

---

model proper (IWM-p), quality-of-thought (Ql Th), and adolescent pregnancy variables, first for the mother cohort and second for the teen cohort. For mothers, the best model of relations among these three variables consisted of 2 two-way effects, Mother's Internal Working Models Proper (Mom's IWM-p) × Mother's Adolescent Pregnancy, and Mother's Internal Working Models Proper (Mom's IWM-p) × Mothers' Quality of Thought, Pearson $\chi^2(6, N = 87), = 10.17, p = .118$. The same two effects constituted the best model for the teen cohort, Pearson $\chi^2(6, N = 87), = 3.88, p = .685$. Odds under these models of the ever-pregnant and never-pregnant outcomes, given internal working models proper, are shown in Table 1, Appendix D. Also shown in this table are the odds of an internal working model classification given an ever-pregnant or never-pregnant status.

[8] A loglinear analysis examined relations among the mother representation (Mom's Rep of Teen), teen working model proper (Teen's IWM-p), and teen adolescent pregnancy

the effects of mothers' representations and teens' working models on teens' pregnancy outcomes are compounding (multiplicative). Having a mother who resentfully depicts daughter as "Daddy's girl" (the BM/GD representation), for example, raises the likelihood of teen pregnancy for daughters with all working models by a factor of 2.2 (the overall odds of pregnancy for daughters of mothers with BM/GD classifications). This compounding produces some marked extremes in the odds of the adolescent pregnancy outcome (8.15 for deprived daughters with mothers who think of them competitively, compared to .09 for mature daughters whose mothers depict both parental relationships positively).

Table 6-4. Odds of Adolescent Pregnancy for Daughters in IWM p x Mother Representation Categories

	Mother Representation Categories			
	MM/BD	BM/GD	GM/GD	Overall
Internal Model				
Deprived	5.81	8.15	1.18	4.20
Competitive	1.80	2.68	.39	1.30
Mature	.48	.68	.09	.33
Overall	1.55	2.20	.32	

Note. MM/BD = Mixed Mom/Bad Dad; BM/GD = Bad Mom/Good Dad; GM/GD = Good Mom/Good Dad.

Other analyses examined whether Mom's IWM-p, quality of thought (Mom's QL TH), or pregnancy status raised or lowered the odds of teens' pregnancies compared to what would be expected from Mom's Rep of Teen alone. The answer to this question in each case was negative.

In sum, those dyads with models suggesting the most difficulty negotiating a path toward psychic maturity are also those in which daughters have been more likely to become pregnant and bear children as unwed adolescents. The effect of daughters' own working models proper on their pregnancy outcomes is compounded by mothers' representations of daughters' relationships, with those mothers who believe that daughters had or currently have a better relationship with fathers than with themselves most likely to have adolescent mothers for daughters.

---

variables. The preferred model of these relations included 2 two-way effects; Mothers' Representations x Teens' pregnancy, and Teens' Internal Working Models × Teens' Pregnancy, Pearson $\chi^2(8, N = 174) = 11.87, p = .157$. Odds of a teen pregnancy expected under the preferred model are shown in Table 6-4.

Generational continuities and discontinuities.[9] Quality-of-thought classifications in the mother and daughter cohorts in our larger sample were unrelated. This is not a surprising finding if we are correct in thinking that quality of thought is particularly susceptible to situational influences such as the level of anxiety of the interviewee, familiarity of the interviewee with the interviewer, or the developmental status of the interviewee.

Generational continuities were found, however, for the working model proper variable. Figure D-1, Appendix D, illustrates this bidirectional relation. On the one hand, mothers' working models proper predicted daughters' working models proper with moderate accuracy (48%, 48%, and 46% concordance in the deprived, competitive, and mature categories, respectively), suggesting that the way a mother unconsciously thinks and feels about her own childhood attachment relationships is somehow communicated to and incorporated by daughter into her own model of relationships. This finding exemplifies what Fraiberg, Adelson, & Shapiro (1975) referred to as the "ghost in the nursery" phenomenon.

On the other hand, mothers of daughters with competitive representations of attachment relationships were especially likely (63%) to also represent their own childhood relationships as competitive. Thus, just as mothers somehow communicate their unconscious relationship conflicts to daughters, so do daughters communicate their unconscious relationship conflicts to mothers. These unconscious communications, it seems,

---

[9] To examine generational continuities, we conducted three loglinear analyses (SPSS–HILOGLINEAR).

The first included the mother and daughter quality-of-thought variables and mothers' representations of daughters. The preferred model emerging from this analysis was constituted by a two-way effect between mothers' quality of thought and their representations of daughters' attachment relationships, Pearson $\chi^2(18, N = 174) = 20.68, p = .296$. The Mother × Teen Quality of Thought effect did not reach significance in tests of partial associations, and it was not included in the preferred model.

The second analysis included mothers' and daughters' internal working models proper and mothers' representations of daughters' attachment relationships. The preferred model included 2 two-way effects—one between mothers' and daughters' working models proper and one between mothers' working models and their representations of daughters' relationships, Pearson $\chi^2(12, N = 174) = 10.62, p = .562$. The two-way partial association between mothers' representations and daughters' working models proper in this analysis was *not* significant, and this effect was not included in the preferred model.

Figure D-1 in Appendix D, section B shows the odds under this model of being a deprived, competitive, or mature daughter given mothers' internal working model classification (D/M) and the odds of being a deprived, competitive, or mature mother given daughters' internal working model classification (M/D).

A third loglinear analysis was performed including Mom's IWM-p, Mom's Ql Th, and Mom's Rep of Teen. All possible two-way interactions were significant (L.R.^{2} (8) = 8.27, p = .677). Figure D-2 in Appendix D, section C shows the odds under the preferred model of the mother representation categories, given mothers' working models proper or quality of thought.

may feed back into mothers' representations of their own childhood attachment relationships.

How mothers represented daughters' attachment relationships (Mom's Rep of Teen) reflected both IWM-p and Mom's Ql TH, but not daughters' own representations of their relationships (Teen's IWM-p). As seen in Figure D-2, Appendix D, Mom's Rep of Teen tended to correspond to Mom's IWM-p—mothers with deprived models tended to view daughters' relationships with both parents as bad, and mothers with mature models tended to view daughters' relationships with both parents as good. The exceptions to this correspondence were competitive mothers who overwhelmingly represented daughters' relationships with themselves as better than with fathers (the Mixed Mom/Bad Dad category). Inasmuch as a significant proportion of competitive mothers had daughters with competitive working models (Figure D-1, Appendix D), these Mixed Mom/Bad Dad representations of daughters' relationships in essence deny daughters' own views of themselves as Daddy's girl. One can speculate that such denial by competitive mothers is an attempt to negate their rivals (fathers) and their daughters' preferences for fathers.

The secure quality of thought for mothers increased the odds (relative to other qualities of thought) that mothers could view both of daughters' parental relationships in a positive light. However, secure mothers, like preoccupied and dismissing mothers, tended most often to have MM/BD representations.

Overall, these findings suggest that mothers' own internal working models proper and qualities of thought act as filters that guide and give shape to their intuitions about daughters' unconscious goals and feelings with respect to parental attachment relationships. Mothers' intuitions about daughters' relationship goals and feelings are no doubt communicated in many subtle ways to daughters through patterns of thoughts, words, feelings, and deeds. Inasmuch as mothers' communications to daughters are important elements of the interactional mix from which daughters construct their own working models, mothers' representations of daughters' relationships can be understood as important components of a process whereby unconscious conflicts are transmitted from generation to generation.

The pattern of generational continuities and discontinuities found in this sample thus point to a view of development as a dialectical process in which changes in mothers' and daughters' models of their own and each others' attachment relationships are ongoing and mutually interdependent. This interdependence is evident both from the interconnections among mother and daughter representational variables and from the bidirectionality of these connections. Findings thus support Erikson's (1963) thesis that mothers and children work together in the shaping and structuring of children's psychic representations and social modalities, or as Loewald (1980) put it, in the negotiation of a path toward psychic maturity.

Relations between quality of thought and internal working models proper. Quality-of-thought and internal working model proper constructs were empirically related in both cohorts. This relation is most evident when subdivisions of the internal working proper variable are maintained in the analysis. Cross-tabulations of frequencies for the quality-of-thought and internal working model proper variables are shown in Table D-2, Appendix D (D).[10]

In both cohorts, secure modes of thinking and talking about internal models were more often associated with competitive and mature than with deprived working models proper. Put somewhat differently, of the two working models proper that might be considered "unfavorable"—competitive and deprived—secure qualities of thought were more often applied to the first than to the second of these models. This finding reinforces the idea proposed in the previous discussion that internal working models proper can be arranged along a developmental continuum and suggests the value of thinking about "unfavorableness" in relative or developmental terms.

In both cohorts, internal working model classifications predicted quality-of-thought classifications more accurately than quality-of-thought classifications predicted internal working model classifications.[11] This difference is consistent with our notion discussed in the beginning of this chapter that working models proper are the bedrock representations that appear temporally prior to qualities of thought and that quality of thought, rather than being synonymous with internal working models, reflects respondents' defensive postures with regard to making information in working models known to self and others in the interview process.

What might be called "favorable" working models proper (mature) were discussed by 39% of mothers and 64% of teens in an insecure manner (preoccupied or dismissing), suggesting that insecurity associated with discussing attachment relationships with an interviewer does not disappear with the advent of more developmentally advanced working models. Whatever the source of this insecurity, it was felt more acutely by mature teens than mature mothers, and particularly so by mature teens whose representations portrayed fathers as shadowy, background figures. The experience of bringing to consciousness thoughts of wanting to become an independent, self-sufficient woman while wanting to remain closely tied to mother produces more anxiety for adolescent girls whose

---

[10] For both cohorts, the two variables were significantly associated, Cramer's $V(10)$ = .54, $p < .01$, for mothers, and Cramer's $V(8) = 26.32$, $p < .001$, for teens.

[11] For mothers, $\lambda = .27$, $T = 2.75$, when IWM-p predicted quality of thought. In contrast, $\lambda = .02$, $T = .19$, when quality of thought predicted IWM-p. Corresponding statistics

fathers are represented as not available for support than for girls whose fathers are represented as playing an important role in their lives.

In sum, empirical relations between working models proper and quality-of-thought constructs suggest that internal working models proper are developmentally ordered and that quality of thought, rather than being synonymous with working models proper, reflects individuals' manner of thinking, feeling, and speaking about them. Adolescents and adults whose models reflect themes and structures characteristic of earlier developmental levels—that is, the deprived and competitive—are those who are most likely to approach the telling of their relationship stories defensively by dismissing the importance of or maintaining an overly preoccupied focus on the details of past and present attachment-related experiences. Inasmuch as defensiveness in the telling implies a wish to avoid something unpleasant, such as a painful or anxious feeling associated with a conscious or unconscious thought or fantasy, this empirical connection between working models proper and quality of thought suggests an interdependence in development between the affective concomitants of underlying representations and developments in their structure and content. Theoretical perspectives on the relation between quality of thought and internal working models proper are discussed in the next chapter.

---

for teens were $\lambda = .32$, $T = 3.17$, when IWM-P predicted quality of thought, and $\lambda = .14$, $T = 1.93$, when quality of thought predicted IWM-p.

7

A Theoretical Framework for Understanding Internal Working Models Proper and Their Relation To Adolescent Pregnancy

The findings in chapters 5 and 6 suggest that girls' sexuality in this African American population is embedded in a complex motivational system that includes both mother and daughter in multiple internalized relations. To say this, however, is not necessarily to believe it unless a theory can be found that pulls together the various threads or themes in a coherent, explanatory system. It is not enough to demonstrate that children, adolescents, and adults vary in their representations of themselves in relationships with attachment figures; that mothers sometimes send daughters mixed messages about their adolescent sexuality; that mothers are involved in their children's psychological development; or that adolescents manifesting higher levels of psychological maturity are more able to resist the unconscious and conscious pulls toward repetition of the adolescent pregnancy behavior pattern than those manifesting lower levels of psychological development. It is also required that we offer an explanation of why these things should be so—an explanation that is internally consistent, logically compelling, sufficiently comprehensive to encompass the full range of things to be explained, and consistent with whatever empirical "facts" are at hand.

A central focus of our explanatory theory, moreover, needs to be on working models proper because this construct has emerged thus far in this work as central to the complex motivational system we seek to explain. Even further, the central focus needs to be on the developmental origins of working models because as Vygotsky (1978) stated, "it is only in movement that a body shows what it is" (pp. 64–65). And as Loewald (1980) said, whereas analyzing a finished product—an extant structure—may give us some insight into its origins, it is only by deriving something from its origins and antecedents that we will ever "understand the unconscious organization and aspects of the human mind, or how where id was, ego may come into being" (p. 210).

Erikson's theoretical descriptions, as I mentioned in the previous chapter, go part of the way toward providing a framework for understanding developments in working models proper. In the remainder of this chapter, I describe two other frameworks that also take a developmental perspective on individuals' mental representations of relationships. The first, the theory from which the internal working model construct per se emerged, is Bowlby's attachment theory as revised by subsequent theorists through the lens of event representation theory. This theory falls short in several ways in accounting for our findings of individual differences in both quality of thought and internal working models proper. The second is Loewald's theory in which mental representational development is framed in the context of the ongoing intrapsychic separation–individuation process motivated by and motivating the eternal conflict between the individual's wish to merge with and to separate from the maternal matrix. This conflict and its developmental vicissitudes is vital to understanding adolescent pregnancy outcomes in this population of poor, African American women.

ATTACHMENT THEORY

Bowlby's Formulations

With the publication in 1985 of "Growing Points of Attachment," a Society for Research in Child Development monograph edited by Bretherton, the construct of internal working models of attachment came into vogue among developmental psychologists and has been making its way into the psychoanalytic literature (e.g., Fonagy, Steele, Moran, Steele, & Higgitt, 1993). The theoretical source of the internal working model construct as discussed in the monograph was Bowlby's attachment theory, which borrowed concepts from ethology, control systems theory, cognitive science, and psychoanalysis. In his tripartite study of attachment, separation, and loss, Bowlby (1969, 1973, 1980) introduced the term *working model* to describe the mental representations that infants, older children, and adolescents construct of themselves in relationships with attachment figures. Implied in his descriptions was the notion that models can differ among individuals along at least three dimensions: thematic contents, or what is represented; structure, or the form in which content is represented; and patterns of behavior or thought about content, particularly patterns of approach toward and/or avoidance of attachment figures, memories and feelings about prior attachment-related events, and expectations and anticipations of future events.

The contents of models, according to Bowlby (1973), include representations of "the [individual's] world and . . . himself in it," including "[the individual's] notions of who his attachment figures are, where they may be found, and how they may be expected to respond," as well as the individual's "notion of how acceptable or unacceptable he himself is in the eyes of his attachment figures" (p. 203). Bowlby believed strongly that these contents derived from experiences individuals have actually had, including their "day to day experiences, . . . statements made to [them] by . . . parents, and . . . information coming from others" (p. 317). Acknowledging the significant role of children's actual experiences with parents in the formation of internal working models corrected what Bowlby considered to be an undue emphasis in prior psychoanalytic accounts on the "role of projection and the individual's own contribution to the misfortunes he experienced" (p. 207).

The structures of models, in Bowlby's account, vary together with goal-corrected attachment plans in complexity and degree of elaboration. The capacity to formulate complex and elaborated models and plans depends, said Bowlby, on the achievement by about age 6 or 7 of what Piaget termed *perspective-taking,* a concrete operational accomplishment occurring together with and implying the waning of egocentrism (Piaget, 1924; Piaget & Inhelder, 1948). To quote Bowlby (1969),

> The truth is that to frame a plan the set-goal of which is to change the set-goal of another's behavior requires a good deal of cognitive and model-building competence. It requires, first, a capacity to attribute to another a capacity to have goals and plans; secondly, an ability to infer from such clues as are given what the other's goals may be; and thirdly, skill in framing a plan that is likely to effect the desired change in the other's set-goal. (p. 352)

With respect to individuals' patterns of thought in relation to attachment, Bowlby suggested that when sources of information used for model construction are compatible, models of parents and self are internally consistent and complementary to one another and children are able to reflect on these models with a degree of accuracy that allows for firm and accurate predictions. Conversely, when information sources conflict, as when the children's own experiences are contradicted by parents' statements, children may adhere to their own viewpoints, thus risking potentially serious ruptures with parents, comply with the parent's version and disown their own, or perhaps try to give credence to both viewpoints by oscillating between them (Bowlby, 1973).

Bowlby, in sum, emphasized the importance of actual experiences and consistencies or inconsistencies therein in both the evolution of model content and patterns of thought in relation to content, as well as the importance of cognitive development as outlined by Piaget in the construction and reconstruction of models. Through these cognitive developmental processes, Bowlby said, models become progressively more structurally sophisticated and complex, and plans for gaining and maintaining proximity to caregivers based on models become progressively more efficient.

Attachment Theorists' Conceptualizations

Individual differences. Attachment theorists (e.g., Bretherton, 1985, 1990, 1991; Grossman, Fremmer-Bombik, Rudolph, & Grossman, 1988; Kobak et al., 1989; Main et al., 1985; Main & Hesse, 1993) have since reconceptualized Bowlby's views about internal working models in terms of event representation theory (Bretherton, 1991; Johnson-Laird, 1983; Nelson, 1983, 1986; Schank, 1982; Schank & Abelson, 1977), a cognitive psychological viewpoint about the nature and development of mental representations. Represented in working models, according to this revised version of Bowlby's theory, are the infant's or child's attempts to gain access to the attachment figure, the attachment figure's response to these attempts: (i.e., to permit access, deny access, or permit it only unpredictably) and the consequent feelings and expectations regarding self and others that emerge from these experiences. As Main et al. (1985) defined them, internal working models are "mental representations of the self in relation to attachment" (p. 67) that are organized out of "experienced outcomes of actions or plans ('intentions') of particular relevance to attachment" (pp. 75–76). Because plans or intentions relevant to attachment are biologically based, largely environmentally stable tendencies to seek to maintain proximity to a central figure (p. 76), possible organizations of caregiver responses, and corresponding major organizations of attachment (internal working models) are finite and limited. These organizations, moreover, capture the basic affective quality of an attachment relationship. That is, "a caregiver may permit access to the infant who seeks proximity (yielding the secure organization), block access (yielding the insecure–avoidant organization), or permit access only unpredictably (yielding the insecure–ambivalent organization)" (p. 76).

In attachment studies, organizational patterns of attachment-related behavior that develop in the 1st year of life are said to be highly resistant to change and predictive of organizational patterns of thought and feelings about attachment at older ages (Bretherton, 1985, 1990, 1991; Fonagy et al., 1991; Main et al., 1985; Ward & Carlson, 1991). These studies collectively suggest, for example, that an avoidant pattern of responding is likely to manifest itself in different forms and through different modalities (behavior, thought, action, feeling) throughout an individual's development. An infant who turns away from or ignores mother after a brief separation in the Strange Situation at age 1 (Ainsworth et al., 1978) may become a preschooler who sidesteps sensitive attachment-related issues on a story-completion task (Bretherton, Prentiss, & Ridgeway, 1990), who may become a 6-year-old who avoids looking at pictures of family members following a brief separation (Main et al., 1985), who may become an adolescent or adult who dismisses the importance of attachment and avoids acknowledging feelings about childhood attachment-related experiences on the AAI (George, Kaplan, & Main, 1985; Main et al., 1985), who may then become a parent whose infant exhibits an avoidant pattern of behavior in the Strange Situation at 1 year of age (Fonagy et al., 1991; Fonagy et al., 1993).

Such stability within individuals is ascribed in attachment studies to environmental stability, to individuals' tendencies to respond to others according to the expectations represented in working models, and to "defensive exclusion" of painful information in working models from conscious awareness. Continuity across generations is attributed to differences among secure and insecure mothers' capacities to respond sensitively to their infants' signals. For example, insecure mothers who tend to avoid their own inner selves are likely to do the same when confronted with their infants' positive or negative affective signals, thereby setting in motion interaction patterns in which infants' attempts or desires to gain access are blocked or granted only unpredictably (Bretherton, 1985, 1990, 1991).

Normative developments. In addition to providing a conceptual basis for understanding what internal working models represent, event representation theory also replaces Piagetian theory in attachment theorists' views as a framework for conceptualizing structural development of models. Citing Stern (1985), Bretherton (1990, 1991) suggested that internal working models begin in early infancy as "registrations" or sensorimotor representations of relatively undifferentiated parent–infant interaction sequences and gradually become reconstructed in more differentiated and integrated forms in an internal plane. Internalized event representations have sequential or syntagmatic structures in which component parts derive meaning from their relation to others in the sequence (Nelson, 1983); that is, they "simulate the spatio-temporal-causal structure of an original experience in connected form" (Bretherton, 1990, p. 276).

Information derived from early, sequentially organized working models is then "reprocessed, partitioned, cross-indexed and summarized" (Bretherton, 1990, p. 276), leading to more structurally complex, hierarchically organized models. For infants, according to Nelson (1983, 1986), events are represented as wholes, not as constructions made up of definable parts. Conceptualizing component parts of scripts (events) as separate, as mental objects that can be manipulated, requires a step of analysis of the script into its parts and the conceptual relations between them. Development in event structures, said Nelson (1983), is essentially a process of "making the implicit (i.e., the structure) explicit (revealing its parts)" (p. 146) and then recombining the differentiated parts in novel ways. In this way, representational development is a process of abstracting paradigmatic conceptual relations from earlier syntagmatic forms.

Normative or age-related developments in the structural and thematic components of working models resulting from this process have been described in work pioneered primarily by Bretherton (e.g., Bretherton, 1991; Bretherton, Prentiss, & Ridgeway, 1990; Watson & Getz, 1990). Her descriptions of normative developments derive from a variety of sources, including studies of the play behavior of infants, toddlers, and preschoolers as well as preschoolers' responses on story-completion tasks. Toddlers, for example, represent simple acts such as sleeping or eating performed on themselves and then more complex sequences of actions including others as actors or recipients (Bretherton, 1984). These representations are dyadic, including mother and self or father and self, but do not include both dyads simultaneously. Preschoolers demonstrate more explicit and differentiated awareness of the structure of routine interpersonal events, allowing for the possibility of substitutions of actors or actions within the same event structure. Older preschoolers include more actions and more actors simultaneously in their representations of attachment-related interactions, represent different roles for themselves vis-à-vis attachment figures (e.g., child, competitor, companion), entertain the idea that multiple roles can be held simultaneously, attribute different roles to mothers and fathers, represent mother and father as having a relationship of their own apart from their respective relationships with the child, and integrate all three dyadic components of the triad in one dynamic structure (Bretherton et al., 1990; Watson & Getz, 1990). These descriptions imply that as children grow older, working models represent selves and others as progressively more internally complex individuals involved in progressively more complex and varied relationships. The correspondence is evident between the normative structural changes in working models described by Bretherton and the structural properties differentiating deprived, competitive, and mature working models proper in this study.

Critique of Attachment Theory

To understand the internal working models proper construct as operationally defined in this study, a theoretical perspective is needed that comprehends the structural and instinctual/affective properties of those models, developmental interrelations between the structural and instinctual/affective components of working models, individual differences among adolescents and adults in both components, the mutual contributions of and interplay between child and adult in model construction, and the particular patterns of relations among mother and daughter representations and adolescent pregnancy demonstrated in the last chapter. In essence, a theory is needed that can adequately describe where the internal worlds reflected in working models proper come from and how they might be related to other internal and external phenomena. For a number of interrelated reasons, attachment theory is not a suitable framework for understanding these aspects of working models.

First, as mentioned previously, adult attachment theorists' one-sided focus on quality of thought to the neglect of the structural or thematic characteristics of working models has led to the erroneous implication in the adult attachment literature that quality of thought and working models are synonymous. Second, although attachment theorists conceptualize the construction of working models as a joint enterprise of child and parent, their narrow focus on infants and children seeking access and caregivers' sensitive or insensitive responses to these attempts omits much that transpires in these joint encounters and that is relevant to an understanding of working models proper, cultural schemas, and the interrelations between them. Third, although attachment theorists include feelings in the list of constituent parts of working models, developmental interrelations between the affective quality of working models and their structural characteristics have not been considered in theoretical or empirical discussions.

Fourth, and perhaps because of the last point, attachment researchers have tentatively approached the possibility of individual differences in the later-developing structural or thematic properties of working models but have not followed up with further theoretical or empirical investigations. For example, Bretherton (1990) described the process whereby working models increase with development in structural complexity as one that would likely result in individual differences among adolescents or adults. From her proposal that ever-more complex models characteristic of preschool and older children develop through a process of differentiation and integration of earlier forms, the assumption follows reasonably that affective and organizational properties of earlier forms would impact subsequent developmental processes. Bretherton (1990) alluded to this idea in the following passage:

> The developmental literature is much less helpful in conceptualizing insecure attachment relationships. It appears that the infant whose signals are consistently ignored or misunderstood does not simply construct an increasingly complex and integrated working model that realistically reflects the interactions of self and others in a mutually unsatisfying attachment relationship. Two processes seem to prevent this. First, the caregiver in such a relationship does not provide sufficient meaningful feedback to the child's signals (possibly on the basis of his or her own distorted working models), and second, defensive processes prevent the child from adequately representing parental insensitivity. This line of reasoning suggests that internal working models developed in insecure attachments not only are less coherently organized from the beginning, *but are also less likely to become more integrated even as metarepresentational processes emerge* [italics added]. (pp. 100–101)

Yet, individual differences in the internal working models of adolescents and adults continue to be conceptualized in the attachment literature in terms of organizational properties apropos to early models of infancy—the latter which are equated with quality of thought—without regard to possible structural differences that may emerge later in development. When Main et al. (1985) defined working models as "the rules for the organization of information relevant to attachment and for obtaining or limiting access to that information," (p. 67) they were referring to these early developing organizational patterns of flexibly accessing, avoiding, or vacillating with respect to thoughts, feelings, and memories about childhood attachment experiences. Through such language and through assessment methods that emphasize quality of thought over content, Main and others implicitly have dismissed the significance of other potentially meaningful structural and thematic individual differences in working models of adolescents or adults.

Fifth, even if we take seriously Bretherton's comment that secure or insecure attachments in infancy can affect subsequent structural developments in models, the direction of effect between quality of thought and internal working models proper implied by her comment would be contradicted by our findings in chapter 6. If quality-of-thought patterns are derivatives of secure or insecure organizational patterns of attachment behavior in infancy and early childhood and if the "security" of an attachment relationship in infancy and early childhood makes a difference with respect to how structural and thematic developments in working models proper subsequently unfold, then we would expect quality of thought to predict internal working model proper classifications with better accuracy than the reverse. On the other hand, if the affective quality of a relationship in infancy and beyond is inextricably interrelated with its structural and thematic components and if quality of thought reflects individuals' defensive postures with regard to bringing these affectively laden, unconscious representations to consciousness in the interview situation, then one would expect working models proper to predict quality of thought with better accuracy than the reverse. As shown in chapter 6, internal working models proper predicted quality of thought in both cohorts better than the reverse.

LOEWALD'S THEORY

An internal working model proper from Loewald's perspective might also be considered a "state of mind," as in Main's formulation, but one that reflects not so much an attentional/representational state as a person's state of mental development. The primary emphasis in Loewald's theory is on development and on mind as an organization of psychic structures and functions that come into being through a lifelong process of internalization. State of mind in that context refers specifically to the degree of internalization characterizing a person's current mental state, reflecting the vicissitudes of his or her developmental history up to the present.

This way of thinking suggests a way of understanding the links observed between internal working models proper and adolescent pregnancies in this population. As reported in the last chapter, women in both cohorts with relatively less internalized models—deprived and competitive—were more likely than those with more internalized models to have been adolescent mothers. Why these inverse relations might hold true awaits further explication of Loewald's views about internalization and what it means in his framework to have a more or less internalized state of mind. First, however, I digress to put Loewald's theory in the broader context of psychoanalytic and developmental theorizing.

Loewald in Context

Hans Loewald (1978, 1980, 1988) was a psychoanalyst whose published writings spanned almost half a century and who, although not well known in the field of developmental psychology, has been recognized among psychoanalysts as "one of the most seminal and influential thinkers in modern psychoanalysis" (Fogel, 1991, p. 4). The central Loewaldian paradox, the one that makes Loewald's views especially suited for interpreting the internal working models described in this study, is that he was at the same time a traditionalist and a radical revisionist of Freud's theory.

As a traditionalist, Loewald retained many classical Freudian concepts, including that of instinct, a notion that Freud (1915) defined early on as a drive—a somatic stimulus impinging on the mind and causing the individual to act in order to reduce or eliminate its effect (the pleasure principle). Although Freud's understanding of instinct underwent many revisions during his lifetime (Compton, 1983), this early definition became and remains the chief focal point of many psychologists' and psychoanalysts' objections to Freudian theory. Psychoanalysts whose theories have had the most impact on developmental psychology, including Bowlby, either discarded or downplayed the so-called Freudian notion of instinct in favor of a view of the individual as active and intrinsically motivated, as seeking to be with and to explore physical and social objects for his or her own sake, and as motivated in this aim by the desire for mastery as well as the biological instinct of survival. Meanwhile, however, the whole range of subjective experiences originally associated with Freud's concept of instinct—affects, urges, wishes, needs—virtually disappeared from theorists' explanations for social and cognitive development. Sroufe and Waters (1977) acknowledged this in pointing to the need to reconceptualize the security motive in Bowlby's and Ainsworth's theories as felt security. Whereas affects now play a larger role in attachment theorists' conceptualizations of the development of secure and insecure patterns of behavior and thought, it remains the case as just mentioned that affective properties of early developing models and later-developing structural properties of models have not been integrated in a theory of development. Although the classical instinct framework within which Loewald situated his views about psychic functioning and development may be somewhat abstract for some readers, it is this framework that offers a vehicle whereby subjective, instinctual/affective experiences can find their way back into developmental theory.

At the same time that Loewald was a traditionalist, he was a radical revisionist of Freud's theory. As such, he recast the notion of instinct within a theoretical framework compatible in key respects with Piaget's and Vygotsky's. In Loewald's (1980) words,

> I have emphasized that as a scientific theory [psychoanalysis] cannot be content to model itself after the traditional scientific theories constructed by such sciences as physics, chemistry or

biology. Their subject matter, as viewed and investigated by these sciences, implies and presupposes a subject–object dichotomy, which is, so to speak, what puts them in business. . . . I have expressed my belief that a theory of the mind, of the psyche as it shows itself to psychoanalytic research, should start with the hypothesis of a psychic matrix within and from which individuation proceeds. . . . I have given a brief account of the processes of internalization and externalization which are involved in individuation and continue to be instrumentalities by which individuation in increasingly complex forms takes its course in human life. I have stressed that what is internalized are dynamic relations between psychic elements of a field of which the internalizing agent is one element. In accord with these views, I reformulated the concept of instinctual drive. (pp. 298–299)

In this passage, Loewald reveals himself as an adherent of the dialectical method. The internal–external dialectic is central in his theorizing, and internalization is proposed as the basic way of functioning of the psyche. In this regard, Loewald's views are compatible with both Piaget's and Vygotsky's ideas about development (Bidell, 1988; Dean, 1994).

The Theory

Loewald's (1980) theoretical writings are about the development of mind, a term that when conceived in relation to the earliest phases of infant development is synonymous with *ego*. As it first comes to be experienced by the very young infant, *ego* does not refer to an agency of the mind to be distinguished from id or superego, but to the first feeling of a difference between the internal and external worlds. The following passage captures the essence of Loewald's views about the early ego and its subsequent development:

> The ego is, as Freud thought—and I believe this is his deepest insight into its psychology—the precipitate, the internalization of what goes on between the primitive psyche and its environment; it is an organization of reproductive action, but action on a new stage, the stage of internality. The interplay on the internal stage of action constitutes the process-structure of the ego. The ego, in its further elaboration and articulation of this reproductive action, which takes place in continuous interaction with the world, then develops toward that more remote, divided, and abstract form of mentation we call the secondary process or representational memory. This mentation is at

the same time more distant and self-divided, and more lucid and free—shall we say sadder and wiser? By virtue of the secondary process, the ego exercises its functions, including that function by which the individual becomes an object of contemplation and care and love in itself and can encounter others as objects in the same spirit. (p. 171)

As in Piaget's (1952) and Vygotsky's (1978) theories, the gradual construction of the ego, of internality, is portrayed by Loewald as a process complementary to the construction of the object world, of externality; each step in one direction implies a complementary step in the other. The internalization process whereby ego and object come into being and are transformed is one in which interactions, regulations, forms of exchange, or relating between subject and object occurring on an external plane are reconstituted in a new form in an internal plane: "Relationships and interactions between the individual psychic apparatus and its environment are changed into inner relationships and interactions within the psychic apparatus" (p. 262).

An insight that links Loewald's perspective to Piaget's is that although internalization is a constructive process of bringing into being an ego world and an object world, it is also a destructive process, in which objects and interactions with them lose their objectivity, lose their object character, and are dissolved and reconstituted as part of the ego. These reconstituted structures thus constitute "psychic representatives" of prior interactions with attachment figures. Loewald (1980) put it this way:

[The] internal world has to be distinguished from the representational world . . . or inner world or "map" . . . constituted by mental representations of objects and their relations to each other. The latter is the secondary or representational memory system; it arises on the basis of the development of the ego and as a function of it. Internalization in the sense intended here is not a process involving the representation of objects and object relations, but it involves, to speak in Freud's language, their dissolution or destruction. In the identifications that may lead to internalization it is precisely the object character of a person that is either not yet established (as in those early identifications preceding object cathexes), or is suspended or annihilated by a process of de-differentiation of subject and object. The object is not represented by the ego to itself, but it becomes deobjectified and depersonifed, and the former object relation becomes a dynamic element of the reorganized ego. (p. 167)

Loewald's theory of development is broadly conceived. It describes not just states of mind and the changes that take place in them, but the process by which these changes occur, the context in which they occur, and the motive forces that propel the ego to pursue its lifelong course of differentiating and integrating. Further, Loewald drew convincing and compelling parallels between all of these facets of so-called normal development and what transpires in the course of a psychoanalysis. The following summary of Loewald's view of development does scant justice to the richness of his conceptions and writings. However, it is sufficient to demonstrate correspondences between the qualitative characteristics of deprived, competitive, and mature working models proper and states of mind characteristic of preoedipal, oedipal, and postoedipal phases of development—correspondences that then merit applying Loewald's explanatory framework in the effort to understand where internal working models proper come from in development and how and why they might be linked to other constructs and behavior patterns of interest in this study.

The preoedipal periods. What is internalized in the beginning, said Loewald (1980), are patterns of excitation coming both from the side of the newborn and the side of the environment. These patterns consist of "incoherent urges, thrashings, and reflex activities" (p. 130) as they are coordinated and organized by the appropriate ministrations of the mother. These ministrations do not necessarily or only reduce or abolish excitation coming from within the infant, but also engender, shape, and organize them, resulting in what Loewald termed alternately the "instinctual activity pattern," "mnemic image," or "mnemic action pattern." In this pattern, "urge and response, environmental engenderment, and the subject's excitation are not differentiated from one another, so that a repetition of such action patterns remains at first a re-enactment of a global event" (p. 131). Loewald (1980) stated,

> In this connection it may be questioned whether the stimulation that becomes psychically represented as instinct can be confined to "inner", organismic stimulation, if "external" stimulation by the mother enters into the formation of instinct. Inasmuch as the entire life of the baby is in the early stages apt to be characterized as instinctual [triebhaft], in response to organic as well as 'external' stimulations, what we call instinctual in psychoanalysis seems at that stage to have more to do with the primitive character of motivation, of psychic organization, than with "organic" versus "environmental." (p. 132)

What for the newborn is at first unorganized and unpatterned becomes organized and patterned through this cycle of internalizing–externalizing activities in which infant and mother are joint participants. Repetitions of global events by the infant are conceived by Loewald not only in the sense of external activity but also in the sense of internal registrations or reverberations of instinctual activity patterns in times of quiescence. The general quiescence of the baby in a state of satisfaction does not mean that psychic activity has ceased. It is more reasonable to assume that "interactions with the world continue to reverberate, are reproduced, and thus lay the foundations for the development of an internal world, in the form of memorial processes" (Loewald, 1980, p. 156). Thus, instinctual activity patterns, like schemes, are a form of memory in that they contain and reproduce the past history of interactions within the infant–mother matrix. They continue or prolong, albeit briefly, for the newborn, the pleasurable experience of undifferentiated oneness with the environment. To use Piaget's (1952) words, they "fill a vaccuum" (p. 141) left by the cessation of activity.

For Loewald, however, repetitions of instinctual activity patterns in times of quiescence are more than just continuations; they are continuations in which something changes. It is here, he said, that the infant's restructuralizing, elaborating, and integrating activities come into play. External interactions are not just retained, but are transmuted—dissolved, destroyed, and reconstituted in a new form, integrated into the total context, thus creating, maintaining, and developing an internal world. How external interactions are restructuralized is a function of the "kind of mind, so to speak, that organizes the material, the fashion and degree of 'schematization' that the mind brings to the material" (Loewald, 1980, pp. 158–159). For the very young infant, these reproduced experiences cannot be anything other than

> quite primitively organized interactions between a primitively organized mind, where a distinction between individual and environment, between memory and what is memorized, is barely in the making, and where sense impressions are likely to be global, all-engulfing and engulfed coenesthetic receptions. (p. 158)

The cycle continues, said Loewald, with the reexternalization of schematized instinctual activity patterns into subsequent interactions within the infant–mother matrix, where they meet with the responsive, caring activity of the mother. The schematization materially influences how the infant perceives and interacts within the infant–mother matrix, "even as new external interactions influence internal reorganization processes by continuing to alter memorial processes" (Loewald, 1980,

p. 162). In a manner very similar to the way in which Vygotsky described the adult's role in the internalization process, Loewald said that the mother, because of her "higher mental development," reflects in her various ministrations and responses "more" than the child presents and helps to give shape and definition to the child's more primitive productions. To quote Loewald (1980),

> The bodily handling of and concern with the child, the manner in which the child is fed, touched, cleaned, the way it is looked at, talked to, called by name, recognized and re-recognized—all these and many other ways of communicating with the child, and communicating to him his identity, sameness, unity and individuality, shape and mould him so that he can begin to identify himself, to feel and recognize himself as one and as separate from others yet with others. The child begins to experience himself as a centered unit by being centered upon. (p. 23)

Through these conjoint organizing activities, the "various elements of action and feeling begin to encounter and know one another; they become a context for meaning" (p. 169). The linking is "no longer merely one of reproductive action; it is one of representational connection" (p. 170). "Insofar as in it duality becomes established, insofar as it differentiates . . . between the perceiver and the perceived" (p. 168), secondary process mentation, equivalent in Loewald's view to "representational memory" (p. 170), thus emerges and branches off from primary process.

There now exists for the child an object, however ill-defined, that is both the source and the recipient of actions, feelings, and urges, as well as a subject (albeit merely a primitive ego-feeling at first), that is likewise the source and recipient of actions, feelings, and urges. To the extent that these psychic fields become increasingly differentiated, there are gains and losses at each new level of organization. On the side of gain, what we think of as "true object relations" or relationships between separate, differentiated people become increasingly possible. On the side of loss,

> becoming an idea means that the unconscious structure loses its unitary, instinctual, "single-minded" character and becomes reinserted into a context of meaning. The loss involved in this transformation is like a death, in that the sadness and grief of mourning involves the giving up of the unitary single-mindedness of instinctual life that tends to preserve in some way the primary narcissistic oneness from which we have to take leave in the development of conscient life and secondary-process mentation. That development involves being split from the embeddedness in an

embracing totality, as well as that internal split by which we come to reflect and confront outselves. The development of conscient, representational memory is a departure from that inner unity and replaces the original unity prior to individuation. Individuation is our human way of memorializing and thus re-creating those origins. (pp. 170–171)

The splitting between perceiver and perceived, self and object, that is the hallmark of secondary process mentation therefore sets in motion the continuing, lifelong effort to resolve the primary conflict inherent in human existence between striving for reunification with the environment (mother) and individuation. It is from this perspective, said Loewald, that the ego's externalizing–internalizing activities must be viewed:

It is the essence of the ego to maintain, at a more and more complex level of differentiation and objectification of reality, this unity in the face of . . . what seems to move further and further away from it and fall into more and more unconnected parts. (pp. 11–12)

At the same time, said Loewald, the unstructured nothingness of identity with the environment represents a threat as deep and frightening as the threat of growing separation and individuation. Thus, "between the danger of a loss of object relationships and the danger of a loss of ego-reality boundaries, the ego pursues its course of integrating reality" (Loewald, 1980, p. 17).

When an infant's internal, experiential object world has differentiated to include the "father figure," the "representative of reality," the latter also takes on an ambivalent status vis-à-vis the ego. On the one hand, the father is an ally in the ego's wish to conserve itself, a figure that reflects the ego's potential for separation and individuation and, as such, a protection against the regressive pull to the state of undifferentiation with the mother. On the other hand, the father figure (reality) constitutes a threat to the developing ego's wish to maintain the original unity with the mother figure. As such, the child is in a defensive relationship vis-à-vis the father.

The Oedipus complex and its resolution. Over time, these ambivalent, preoedipal intrapsychic dyadic relationships with mother and father figures become components of the Oedipus complex, defined by Loewald as a "psychic representation of a central, instinctually motivated, triangular conflictual constellation of child–parent relations" (Loewald, 1980, p. 384). The Oedipus complex is thus heir to developments in the preceding dyadic intrapsychic interactions between child and mother, child and father. Object relations among conceptually distinct individuals become increasingly complex in the oedipal phase as their scope widens to include not just dyads, but child, mother, father, siblings, and other primary attachment figures in triadic and even more complex systems.

Among individual children, adolescents, and adults, the Oedipus complex can be manifested in many shapes and forms depending on the vicissitudes of prior development, current environmental factors, cultural practices, and the like. There is no reason to expect uniformity in this regard among children within the same family, much less among children within or between societies. There is, however, more reason to expect that once children develop a view of themselves as separate and distinct individuals with the capacity to say "no," to oppose their parents' will, and to assert their own will and take initiatives of their own choosing, they will want what they perceive their parents and siblings have that they do not, including special relationships that exclude potential intruders into those relationships. If the desired special relationship is with one parent, the other parent as well as siblings can be viewed as potentially threatening rivals. Although parents may perceive or sense these feelings in their children, under optimal conditions they will refrain from either extreme of gratification or punishment, allowing the child to experience both the desire and defeat, together with associated emotions of love, hostility, and guilt, in a context of relative safety and support.

The manner in which the Oedipus complex is resolved, in which the child handles the conflicts inherent in the Oedipus complex, will impact the course of his or her future development. One way is by repression, which is "an unconscious evasion of the emancipatory murder of the parents, and a way of preserving infantile libidinal-dependent ties with them" (Loewald, 1980, p. 390). Another is by "destruction" or "parricide," which is

> carried out in that dual activity in which aspects of oedipal relations are transformed into ego–superego relations (internalization), and other aspects are, qua relations with external objects, restructured in such a way that the incestuous character of object relations gives way to novel forms of object choice. These novel object choices are under the influence of those internalizations. Insofar as human beings strive for emancipation and individuation as well as for object love, parricide on the plane of psychic action is a developmental necessity. (p. 390)

Thus,

> emancipation as a process of separation from external objects—
> to be distinguished from rebellion, which maintains the external

relationship—goes hand in hand with the work of internalization, which reduces or abolishes the sense of external deprivation
and loss. Whether separation from a love object is experienced
as deprivation and loss or as emancipation and mastery will
depend, in part, on the achievement of the work of internalization. (p. 263)

To the extent that internalization of oedipal object relations is completed,

the individual is enriched by the relationship he has had with the
beloved object, not burdened by identification and fantasy relations with the object. We are most familiar with th(is) transformation . . . from the development of the child's love attachments
to his parents into the adult's mature heterosexual love relationships, a development that includes oedipal object relinquishment
and internalization, freeing the individual for non-incestuous
object relations. This freedom is not simply freedom from old
object ties that have been cast off, but an inner freedom we call
maturity, achieved by internalization of old ties. (p. 83)

Adolescence and beyond. No matter how resolutely or by what process
the ego masters the Oedipus complex in its original action, said Loewald,
it returns in adolescence and in later periods of life for so-called normal
people and neurotics and repeatedly requires some form of mastery. At
this phase, superego structures undergo fresh phases of disorganization,
involving reexternalization and deneutralization of previously internalized instinctual components. In adolescence, spontaneous, intrapsychic
oedipal involvements are partially relinquished and transformed again so
that individual and new involvements can proceed, a process "facilitated
and promoted by parental instinctual disengagement" (Loewald, 1980,
p. 311). Seen in this light, said Loewald, "there is no definitive destruction of the Oedipus complex, even when it is more than repressed; but we
can speak of its waning and the various forms in which this occurs"
(p. 311).

The dependence–emancipation struggles in adolescence, Loewald
(1980) suggested, are something more than symbolic action. They are

palpable factual experiences that may and do in the end diminish one side or the other. Parents or children tend to be rendered
relatively impotent, at least as far as the generational engagement
is concerned. Parricide, if the child convincingly develops as an
individual, is more than symbolic or on the plane of intrapsychic

reorganization. In our role as children of our parents, by genuine emancipation we do kill something vital in them—not all in one blow and not in all respects, but contributing to their dying. As parents of our children, we undergo the same fate, unless we diminish them. If eventually some sort of balance, equality, or transcending conciliation is achieved, children and parents are fortunate. It is a balance or harmony that in the external no less the internal arena remains vulnerable . . . and requires continued internal activity. (p. 395)

Beyond adolescence, new integrative tasks in life, imposed by changing life circumstances or chosen by creative individuals, tend to trigger such reactivations. Loewald suggested that this may reflect a healthy resiliency of the ego, which enables the individual to engage in a disorganization in the service of the ego—"to undo, to an extent, former structural resolutions to arrive at novel resolutions, at higher levels of organization" (Loewald, 1980, p. 340).

Summary

To summarize, Loewald viewed the development of mind as a process of progressive differentiations and integrations of psychic structures and functions that continues throughout a person's lifetime except when blocked by neurosis or psychosis. Differentiations and integrations come about through internalization, or the reconstitution in the internal plane of interactions occurring first on an external plane. Internalization, therefore, always takes place in the context of a matrix involving the individual and others who are of primary emotional significance. These others and the individual conjointly construct, define, and direct the pathway of development.

At the same time that internal structure comes into being and is continually reorganized on an internal plane, changes take place in the relation between internality and externality, or in the intrapsychic relation between the ego and external objects. From a state of initial undifferentiation of inner and outer comes a state of awareness that some sources of stimulation have an external source and others an internal source. This state of awareness is at best incomplete at first. Gradually through cycles of internalizations and externalizations, mother and infant give shape and definition to these various sources of stimulation so that the child can differentiate not only self from mother but mother from father, siblings, and perhaps other important attachment figures. True object relations between differentiated objects are now possible and lead into the central, instinctually motivated, triangular conflictual constellation of parent–child relations known as the Oedipus complex. Resolution of the complex by "parricide" on the level of psychic action destroys or de-differentiates object relations in the sense that they are integrated as part of the ego–superego and lose their instinctual, incestuous character.

Child and adult participate together in the internalizing–externalizing cycle not only because they are biological organisms striving for progressively higher forms of adaptation, but also because they have a personal need to resolve ongoing instinctual/affective conflicts between individuation and reunion with the environment that originate in the splitting of primary process mentation into perceiver and perceived. At each developmental step, the conflict arises in new form, determined as Erikson (1963) indicated, by what the infant or child is inherently equipped and predisposed to do, what the infant or child has learned to do and has constructed for herself, and what the mother and society expect and either encourage or discourage the child to do. By internalizing interactions within the child–adult matrix, the child simultaneously preserves and enriches psychic structure, develops more powerful means of keeping the object within his or her scope, and makes these interactions a part of his or her internal structure, thus maintaining unity on a symbolic level. To the extent that individuation is experienced as a loss, the primary conflict is reinstated and the cycle continues. Thus, the subjective, instinctual/affective experiences of the two participants, in Loewald's viewpoint, both motivate and are motivated by the internalization process.

Internal Working Models Proper

In Loewald's perspective, then, internal working models proper are states of mind in the sense that they reflect different degrees of internalization or states of mental development. The deprived model captures a range of states characterized by relatively less differentiation between internality and externality. The competitive model subsumes a range of more differentiated states of mind, but in which childhood attachment figures remain the primary intrapsychic focus. The progress of internalization is manifested in mature models by the de-differentiation of ego from primary attachment objects—that is, the integration of interactions and relationships with these objects into the ego–superego structure and the concomitant shifting of instinctual interests to others outside the "womb of the family" (Erikson, 1963, p. 259).

These different manifestations of states of mind, these variations among child–adult dyads in their success in negotiating a path toward psychic maturity, are understood by Loewald as a function of individual variations in the quality of the instinctual/affective bond. As he put it, "disturbances of internalizing and externalizing processes, caused by deficiencies—for whatever reason—in the vicissitudes of attunement between child and human environment, spell disturbance of individuation, of psychic-structure formation" (p. 212).

Ideally, said Loewald, a parent is in an empathic relation to the child. At the same time that he or she presents to the child a more organized, articulated view of the child's core of being, thus mediating a vision of what the child can become, the parent meets the child at the child's own level. For the child to identify with or internalize the parent's more articulate image, that image must be recognizable to the child as a reflection of him- or herself. The creation by the parents of this optimal environment, this sliding balance, said Loewald, is not merely in the interest of the child's development but represents a developmental change in the parents. They progressively loosen the libidinized or aggressivized ties with the child as their external object, leading to "further internalization processes in themselves and modification of their own ego structures" (p. 267).

Parents, however, never attain the ideal in reality, but only approximate it to greater or lesser degrees depending largely on their own success in negotiating a course between the two poles of the primary conflict. The particular links of meaning among action, urge, and feeling that are mediated by the parents' response and transmuted into internal structure profoundly influence the child's image of self in relation to the environment. This image affects whether the child strives more for individuation, reunification, or balance, imbuing the internalization process with a particular emotional significance that may be retained through life.

The current state of mind of an adult or adolescent implies an intrapsychic history that cannot be ascertained from a single interview. Models reflecting the deprived and competitive states do not necessarily imply that individuals remain stuck in the same states of mind they had as infants or young children. Adolescence, as Loewald suggested, is a time when what has been internalized tends to be reexternalized, opening up possibilities for reorganization. This is also the case at critical times in later life phases. Thus, it is not possible to know with certainty whether deprived and competitive models of adolescent or adults in this study reflect a reexternalization of something that was previously internalized, whether there has been a slowdown or relative arrest in the internalization process. The very question, however, raises the possibility of reorganization of attachment representations for individuals of all ages.

Internal Working Models and Adolescent Pregnancy

By putting individual differences in the thematic and structural characteristics of working models proper in the broader context of the ongoing process of intrapsychic separation and individuation, Loewald's internalization theory helps to clarify why the probabilities of adolescent pregnancy vary with the developmental status of working models proper. I have suggested that the characteristics of deprived, competitive, and mature working models proper correspond generally to the characteristics of mental states in preoedipal, oedipal, and postoedipal phases of development, respectively. These characteristics are evident in women's behavioral and verbal modes of expressing unconscious fantasies or sets of unconscious beliefs about themselves in relationships with others, including those aspects pertaining to wanting, having, conceiving, bearing, giving, or being babies. From what has been said thus far about Loewald's views about development, four dimensions can be identified on which the progress of internalization can be gauged, on which internal working models proper can be differentiated, and which have implications for adolescent pregnancy. Although I have distinguished these dimensions for the sake of discussion, it will be clear in that discussion that the four dimensions are several sides of the same coin.

Blurring and blending of internal and external objects and events. First, one gauge of the progress of internalization according to Loewald's descriptions are degrees of intrapsychic differentiation between what comes from within and what comes from without. Relatively less differentiation is characteristic of deprived models, as compared with competitive or mature, although it is the case that some degree of blurring and blending characterizes all states of mental development. Deprived models reflect a mental state in which object and ego are intertwined in a way not seen in higher level models, in which confusions are rampant regarding whose mental products (thoughts, feelings, needs, wishes) are whose.

One version of the core unconscious fantasy characteristic of deprived models inferred from interviews and conversations reflects these confusions and goes something like this. A girl wants and needs the kind of warmth and comfort that only mothers can provide for their babies, but feels was not forthcoming when she was a baby or later in her life. This kind of relationship with mother was and is intensely desired and missed. One belief, therefore, is that mother did not and does not love her—that mother was and maybe still is depriving. This belief, however, blends easily and quickly into the thought that it is mother who was deprived of a baby she could love and who would love her in return, a baby more satisfactory than the girl herself. Mother is someone who would have loved daughter if she had been the kind of baby mother wanted. Conceiving a baby of her own and loving it, while giving it to or sharing it with mother, is one way out of this dilemma to the extent that daughter, in her unconscious fantasy, can identify herself with baby. Being baby or identified with baby on a symbolic level provides the girl an opportunity to mother herself in the way she has yearned for throughout her life, for mother to mother her in that way as well, and for mother to love her for giving her the baby mother has always wanted.

At the same time that a girl with a deprived model fantasizes ways to re-create and maintain close connections with mother, however, mother is believed to be a dangerous person with whom to be in a close relationship. In conversations and interview narratives, women's expressed yearnings of closeness and warmth with mother led frequently into dangerous territory, into memories of mother as abusive, uncaring, unfeeling, and rejecting. In this regard, having a baby can be a way to distance oneself from mother, to individuate, by having something that mother no longer has, by becoming an adult on more equal footing with mother.[1]

Whereas not all fantasies of deprived women in this study contained all of these elements or were put together in this same way, at least some of the component beliefs could be heard in every story. These component beliefs are (a) that mothers can provide intensely desired and sorely missed warmth and comfort that babies should get from their mothers but at the same time can inflict emotional and physical pain and suffering on daughters if they get too close or too dependent, (b) that what mothers want and have always wanted is a baby, (c) that they (daughters) themselves were not satisfactory babies, (d) that mothers love babies more than grown-up children, (e) that if grown-up children were babies they would be loved more, and (f) or that if grown-up children give mother a baby they will be loved more. In these beliefs and the overarching storyline that ties them together, there is an implicit blurring and blending of mother's

---

[1] Blos (1962) described two types of "female delinquents," by which he meant girls who act out sexually as adolescents. One type "has regressed to the preoedipal mother," the other "clings desperately to a foothold on the oedipal stage" (p. 234). This description of the "core" underlying fantasy of girls with deprived models resembles Blos's description of the first type. As Blos described it,

> The delinquent girl who has failed in her liberation from the mother protects herself against regression by a wild display of pseudoheterosexuality. . . . The pseudo-heterosexuality of this type of delinquent girl serves as a defense against the regressive pull to the preoedipal mother. . . . An acute disappointment in the mother is frequently the decisive precipitating factor in illegitimacy. By proxy the mother–child unit becomes re-established, but under the most foreboding circumstances for the child. Unwed mothers of this type can find satisfaction in motherhood only as long as the infant is dependent upon them; they turn against the child as soon as independent striving asserts itself. Infantilization of the child is the result. (pp. 236–237)

needs with the girl's own needs and of her identity as a grown-up child with her identity as a baby.

In keeping with Loewald's descriptions of "instinctual activity patterns" as reflecting both inner, organismic stimulation and external stimulation by the mother, the set of unconscious beliefs constituting the deprived model can also be understood as a joint construction of mother and daughter in which respective contributions are not clearly differentiated. For example, the belief that mother wants a baby may derive in part from a girl's correct reading of mother's implicit messages regarding the desired outcome of her adolescent sexual activity as well as from daughter's projection onto mother of her own wish to have a baby for reasons just mentioned, or from other reasons. Daughter's belief that she was not a satisfactory baby and is not a satisfactory adolescent child may derive in part from mother's implicit or explicit rejection of her and from her own sense of badness stemming from unconscionable unconscious wishes and feelings. Daughter's belief that she and mother can have another try at a close, loving relationship through the insertion of a new baby in the equation may reflect both mother's and daughter's undistinguished wishes.

Daughters with such relatively undifferentiated states of mind may be particularly susceptible to mothers' implicit and explicit messages because these messages may be felt at some level of mind as daughters' own. This difficulty distinguishing whose mental products are whose may reflect compatibility between mothers' and daughters' mental products and it may also reflect both parties' defensive reactions to the dangers associated with being differentiated and separate people. In contrast, mothers and adolescent daughters who are able to relate to one another from intrapsychic positions of greater differentiation, equality, and mutual respect—for example, those with mature and competitive working models proper - might be more able to recognize, tolerate, and acknowledge differences in underlying goals and means for achieving them. In the next chapter, this general question is addressed empirically in the specific context of examining whether mothers' implicit messages about adolescent sexuality have more impact on behavioral outcomes for daughters with deprived than competitive or mature models.

Action versus thought as a mode of instinctual/affective expression.
Second, Loewald, like Piaget, suggested that developmentally earlier states of mind tend toward the enactive versus mental representational mode of psychic representing. Mother and infant relate to each other through cycles of internalizing–externalizing activities in which both are joint participants. For the young infant, repetitions of instinctual activity patterns, both externally and internally in the form of registrations or reverberations, are means of keeping mother within the infant's scope, of prolonging the experience

of undifferentiated oneness with the environment, of filling a vacuum left by the cessation of activity.

In infant development, said Loewald, repetitions of these patterns internally are not just continuations, but repetitions in which something changes, in which shape and definition is given through restructuring by the infant and through the ministrations of the mother. As the duality of inner and outer that is the hallmark of secondary process thought becomes progressively more distinct through this joint process, mental representational thought in the sense of ideas and images more and more binds action (i.e., contains it internally). Mental representation supplements and supersedes action as a means of keeping mother within the child's scope.

Ultimately, said Loewald, this function served by the mental re-presentation of the object to the ego is superseded in development, if things go well enough, by the symbolic destruction of the object per se and the integration of interactions with the object as components of the ego–superego internalized structure. Thus, what we have in good enough development is a shift in primary modes of relating and maintaining contact with attachment figures from repetitions of instinctual activity patterns, to mental representation, to integration of object relationships as part of the ego.

This gauge of the progress of internalization is a second way of characterizing differences between working models proper and understanding the adolescent pregnancy behavior pattern. There are two ways in which it could be said that women with deprived and competitive models enact or repeat activity patterns to a greater extent than women with mature models, both of which could be viewed as defensive means of keeping an attachment figure with the ego's scope, of holding onto a relationship that threatens to dissolve, to be disrupted, or to be torn away.

One way is by incessant repetitions both in behavior and thought of sado-masochistic interactions with mother, interactions involving mutual exploitation, power struggles, competitions, and never-ending efforts to extract scarce emotional and material supplies from the other. For women with deprived and competitive models, these are familiar modes of interacting that have been in place since childhood. Their repetition on external and/or internal planes may serve unconsciously, as Coen (1992) suggested, as a means of binding self to mother, of re-creating her presence through familiar interactions, while avoiding the two worse fates of total destruction of the relationship or transformation of the relationship into one of true intimacy. In Loewald's perspective, these seemingly endless sado-masochistic engagements may be the ego's solution to the dangers posed by individuation on the one hand and merger on the other.

A second way has been suggested by Main (1995) in her descriptions of the organized, insecure, preoccupied, and dismissing states of mind or qualities of thought used relatively more often by women with deprived and competitive working models proper. These qualities of thought, Main said, are aimed at maintaining a "steady attentional/representational state" in the face of remembered inconsistencies and rejections from attachment figures and transferred expectations of the same from an interviewer. The insecure organized qualities are repeated action patterns in which nothing changes. As Loewald described in relation to infant development, they do not meet with the responsive, caring activity of the mother who, because of her higher mental development, can reflect "more" than the respondent presents and can help to give shape and definition to her productions. They are action patterns in which nothing changes because the "kind of mind" that organizes them believes unconsciously that the exact repetition of these patterns is necessary for both the continuation of the relationship and the preservation of self as at least a semi-individuated person.

A greater possibility exists, however, for women with the competitive model rather than the deprived model of recognizing, describing, and reflecting insightfully on both interactions with mother and cognitive action patterns used defensively to maintain ties with her. This difference is evident in the percentages of deprived (17%) versus competitive (37%) women who exhibited the secure quality of thought. Women who used the secure quality of thought demonstrated that it is possible to develop an observing ego, to separate the "observing" part of the ego from what is observed within, to sustain that duality that implies "mental representation" in the sense of a creation that presents internal and external events to the mind. Women with the more differentiated competitive model have an advantage in this regard over women with less differentiated deprived models. However, although percentages are small, the data just reported suggest that it is possible for individuals with deprived models to recognize, acknowledge, and reflect on the confusion that has existed and may still exist in their minds about what thoughts and feelings belong to them or to others and to reflect on the defensive purposes of such confusions as well as the underlying fears that necessitate the defense.

In this context, the act of becoming pregnant as an adolescent can be seen in part as a by-product of the general tendency of women with less internalized models to enact patterns of relationships rather than to represent them internally. Further, such acts can be seen as serving the same functions of maintaining ties while keeping distance as are manifested in sado-masochistic interactional exchanges and organized insecure qualities of thought . A tendency toward action as a mode of expression translates beliefs that comprise unconscious fantasies into behavior rather than into thoughts that can be verbalized to oneself or to others and, in so doing, become reshaped and redefined.

Thematic content. A third gauge of the progress of internalization indicated in Loewald's descriptions of development is the content of a person's unconscious thoughts—that is, what the person wants in interactions with primary attachment figures, how a person might go about getting what she wants, and what she anticipates will happen as a result of wanting and trying to get what she wants. Having a baby as an adolescent, with all the attendant meanings this act has for the girl's intrapsychic and interpersonal relationship with mother, fits in well with the core fantasies of girls with deprived and competitive models but not with those of women with mature models. Previously, I described a set of beliefs that are components of the core unconscious fantasy defining the deprived model. Generally speaking, these beliefs are organized around the two goals of forging and maintaining a connection with mother while keeping sufficient emotional distance and self-integrity to protect from the destructive tendencies of both mother and self. Having, sharing, and/or giving a baby to mother has a definite role in this fantasy and can be used in the service of both objectives.

The same two goals are evident in the contents of both competitive and mature respondents' narratives but are manifested in different unconscious core fantasies. Having a baby as an adolescent and giving it to or sharing it with mother has a place in the competitive model fantasy but not the mature. The unconscious wishes and beliefs that constitute the competitive model core fantasy are that daughter is mother's competitor for father's love and affection, that father loves daughter more than mother; that daughter can have father's baby, and that mother is angry with and jealous of daughter because of father's preference for her and because of mother's own desire for a new baby. Coinciding with these beliefs are another set in which father is thought of as frustrating and disloyal, whereas mother is desired as a person who can provide daughter with needed love, affection, support, advice, and instruction about life and about being a woman. Thus, a girl's unconscious wish or belief that she can have a baby with father, with the baby's actual father standing in symbolically for father, represents a victory over mother. In turn, by giving baby to or sharing baby with mother, the girl can atone for the perceived damage and hurt inflicted on mother. The baby a girl may have, then, represents both victory and atonement.[2]

---

[2] Blos (1962), in describing the second type of female delinquent—the type that comes closest to women in this study with competitive models—said the following:

This second type of delinquent girl has not only experienced an oedipal defeat at the hands of a—literally or figuratively—distant, cruel or absent father, but, in addition has also witnessed her mother's dissatisfaction with her husband; mother and daughter share their disappointment and a strong and highly ambivalent bond continues to exist between them. Under these circumstances, no satisfactory identi-

The unconscious wishes and beliefs that characterize the mature model core fantasy are that mother and father are human beings with some qualities that are admirable and others that may not be so admirable. They are human beings who have strengths, weaknesses, and problems and who have coped with problems in ways that have met with varying degrees of success. They are mentors who, to the extent possible, have given of themselves, their advice, their love, in an effort to provide daughter with the knowledge and personality characteristics she will need to make her way in the world without them. An important wish or belief in this fantasy is that by being like mother in ways that are admired, daughter can be with her symbolically while being away from her, being different and independent. Having a baby as an adolescent symbolically for mother or with father has no place in the context of this fantasy but will have a place in the context of a relationship with a man who belongs to her and not to her mother.

De-differentiation of internal and external. A fourth gauge of the progress of internalization is the degree to which relationships with primary attachment figures fantasied as part of the Oedipus complex are destroyed, dissolved, or transmuted and reconstituted into components of the ego–superego internal psychic structure. In other words, the question here is, to what degree has a person relinquished the intrapsychic fantasy of deriving instinctual gratifications from primary, childhood attachment figures in favor of attempting to do the same in the context of new relationships "outside the womb of the family" (Erikson, 1963, p. 259)? Either women in this study with mature models have progressed further in this regard than those with competitive or deprived, or those with competitive or deprived models have reexternalized their unconscious fantasies back into the realm of interactions with primary attachment figures.

Everything that has been said thus far points to the conclusion that less "emancipated" girls are more likely than others to desire babies at an age and in circumstances intimately involving mother and/or father in the symbolic conception or upbringing of the child. Further, the implicit message from mothers that adolescent pregnancy is a desired outcome is likely

---

fication with mother can be achieved; instead a hostile or negative identification forges a destructive and indestructible relationship between mother and daughter. Young adolescent girls of this type quite consciously fantasy that if only they could be in their mother's place the father would show his true self, that he would be transfigured by their love into the man of their oedipal wishes. . . . In more general terms we may say that her delinquent behavior is motivated by the girl's need for the constant possession of a partner who serves her to surmount in fantasy an oedipal impasse— but more important than this, to take revenge on the mother who had hated, rejected, or ridiculed father. (p. 235)

to be more compelling not only for girls whose self-representations are less differentiated from representations of mothers (deprived models), but also for girls whose affective energies remain invested in intrapsychic relationships with primary attachment figures (deprived and competitive representations).

Quality of Thought

Loewald's views contribute both to an understanding of internal working models proper and to a conceptualization of the quality-of-thought construct and its relation to internal working models proper. This conceptualization is close to Main's (1995) most recent formulation of the internal working model or state of mind construct operationalized in her scheme for coding the AAI. It must be emphasized again, however, that parallels at a conceptual level do not translate into comparability of different empirical measures of the construct. The extent to which similar findings would be obtained using our methods for assessing quality of thought, on the one hand, and Main's coding scheme, on the other, is an empirical question that can only be answered by further research. Regardless of the overlap in meaning, the findings of this study cannot speak directly to those in other attachment studies, but they can and do raise questions and possibilities that could be pursued in further studies.

Main's (1995) most recent formulation is that insecure organized states of mind about attachment as manifested on the AAI are attentional/representational states adopted as means of maintaining a connection while protecting self from anticipated painful aspects of memories of primary attachment relationships. These states adopted in the interview situation parallel and may derive directly from states manifested in infants' patterns of behavior vis-à-vis primary attachment figures. Thus, states of mind are postures adopted in relation to an important other person that have both adaptational and defensive aspects. The adaptational aspect is that which maintains the connection, and the defensive aspect is that which protects from painful feelings and other consequences.

The view of the quality-of-thought construct that I have put forth in this study is in basic agreement with Main's formulation. However, in contrast to Main, who applied this description to organized insecure but not secure or disorganized states of mind, I argue in keeping with Loewald's (1980) views that all states of mind or qualities of thought serve the same two functions of adaptation and defense. The secure quality of thought serves the function of defense inasmuch as open acknowledgement and reflection on attachment-related memories and issues can in itself bring about relief from suffering, and it serves the function of adaptation inasmuch as the latter can lead to further internalization, growth, intrapsychic separation, and individuation—the capacity to form new potentially more healthy and satisfying relationships. Likewise, the disorganized state of mind ultimately maintains the connection and protects through a temporary break in the connection.

These differing postures are taken in relation to something else, which in this study I have termed internal working models proper. This something else is not an external object per se, but the unconscious representation of self in relationships with external objects. It is a representation with predominant themes reflecting predominant instinctual wishes and modes of gratifying them, beliefs about self and others that are associated with those wishes, and structural characteristics reflecting degrees of differentiation, integration, neutralization, and the like—all of which reflect a state of development or degree of internalization. Internal working models proper as so conceptualized are distinct from quality of thought, or postures taken in relation to them, both conceptually and empirically, as was demonstrated and discussed in chapter 4. Making this distinction and measuring the two constructs separately are essential for understanding adolescent pregnancy in this poor, African American population.

Internalization in the Larger Sociocultural Context

Although Loewald's theory as presented in this chapter focuses more on the individual (infant–mother, child–adult) end of the contextual spectrum, aspects of it are also applicable to an understanding of the relations of individuals to the larger society of which they are a part and thus to an understanding of the adolescent pregnancy system as a whole. The internalizing–externalizing cycles that Loewald described occur in ever-widening contexts—the infant–mother, child–adult, adult–society matrices. It is in these contexts that the internal and external worlds meet, mix, distill, and are then reinternalized. Further, internalization theory views child and adult, individual, and society as joint participants in a dialectical process in which both are in a constant state of development and change. These generalizations of Loewald's theory into the individual–society matrix are pursued in more detail in chapters 8 and 9.

8

Putting Culture and Psyche Together with Adolescent Pregnancy

Thus far in this book, some cultural and personal themes in the adolescent pregnancy "symphony" have been identified. We have seen how both cultural and personal themes play out within and between mother and daughter cohorts, and we have seen how both categories of themes relate individually to mothers' and daughters' adolescent pregnancy outcomes. Cultural themes suggested that adolescent pregnancies have served important functions for poor African Americans in the past and continue to do so in the present, especially in downwardly mobile and traditional family environments; that many mothers in these family contexts have internalized cultural schemas in which adolescent pregnancy is represented as a desirable outcome; that this message is communicated unknowingly and unwittingly to daughters through inconsistencies in their emotional productions, words, and deeds; and that some daughters act on these messages by becoming pregnant as unwed adolescents. Daughters' actions of becoming pregnant or not as adolescents enter into the construction of their own cultural schemas, which then become the basis for further communications to the next generation of adolescent girls.

Rather than closing the book on our investigation of the adolescent pregnancy phenomenon in this population, however, these findings take us back to theoretical questions raised in the introduction. There, we made reference to an ongoing debate of concern to both cultural anthropologists and psychologists over whether it is necessary to invoke both individual psychological and cultural constructs in explaining socially significant action patterns such as adolescent pregnancies. Some theorists argue that psychological and cultural sources of motivation are distinct and interacting (e.g., LeVine, 1982; Spiro, 1961), others argue that the two are indistinguishable or that one supersedes the other (e.g., Shweder & Sullivan, 1990), whereas still others argue that cultural and psychological forces are interdependent poles of irreducible wholes that contain within them the essential conditions for change (e.g., Bretherton, 1985; D'Andrade, 1990; Loewald, 1980).

Almost by definition, the cultural schemas identified in chapter 5 contradict the idea that cultural and psychological sources of motivation are separate and distinct. The schemas manifested by mothers through combinations of emotional displays, words, and deeds, whether consistent or inconsistent, are both cultural and psychological; they belong to both individual and collective minds. Many girls interviewed in this phase of our study thought, felt, and behaved in accordance with what they perceived their mothers wanted in regard to their adolescent sexuality. In turn, mothers' wants reflected their perceptions of social and economic pressures and opportunities emanating from family environments and experiences as adolescent mothers and from their perceptions of what their own mothers wanted. Mothers are thus representatives of the collective mind and vehicles whereby cultural messages are communicated to future generations of individuals. When seen from this perspective, cultural and psychological, collective and individual blend together in barely distinguishable form.

The question remained after chapter 5, however, as to the need to search for additional, more personal sources of motivation for adolescent sexual behavior and pregnancies. Is it the case, as Shweder argued, that "behavior follows the curves of culturally defined realities and no other forces (of material interests or repressed needs) are required to explain why we do what we do" (as cited in Strauss, 1992, p. 13)? Or is it the case, as those with dialectical viewpoints would argue, that those "other forces" constitute an indispensable pole in an individual–social relation that is necessary to explain both individuals' responses to cultural messages and the possibilities for change in the adolescent pregnancy behavior system?

The hypothesis put forth in this book has been that other forces *are* required to explain why individuals do what they do. Whereas the findings in chapter 5 emphasized the importance of mothers' adolescent pregnancy histories and family environments for their cultural schemas and the importance of family enviroment for daughters' adolescent pregnancy outcomes, the findings also pointed to the likelihood of other sources of variability for both schemas and pregnancy outcomes. Some daughters of mothers with inconsistent cultural schemas, for example, held attitudes and beliefs about adolescent pregnancy that were clearly contrary to mothers', and some daughters whose mothers communicated mixed messages had not yet become pregnant. Further, some women who had become mothers as adolescents and who had grown up in downwardly mobile or traditional families—contexts in which inconsistent cultural schemas predominate—were consistent in both their implicit and explicit opposition to daughters' potential adolescent pregnancies. Other forces may enter into the adolescent pregnancy picture both directly and as factors in why some mothers resist the construction of schemas implicitly encouraging pregnancy or in why some daughters more than others internalize the meanings of cultural messages conveyed by mothers as their own thoughts, feelings, and prescriptions for action.

The direct effects of other forces implicated in the adolescent pregnancy system—that is, personal representations including working models proper and quality of thought—were the focus of our investigations in chapter 6. In that chapter, we took the first step in examining the part played by women's working models of their own or their daughters' attachment relationships by identifying and interpreting patterns in both the content and quality of thought exhibited in discourse about those relationships. Quantitative analyses of relations among quality-of-thought and internal working model proper constructs within and across cohorts, and between the latter and adolescent pregnancy, suggested a prominent role for internal working models proper in the adolescent pregnancy system.

Goals of This Chapter

The task remaining in this chapter is to see how personal and cultural themes go together and work together in the process of maintaining or interrupting the adolescent pregnancy behavior pattern. In the first section, I focus on direct empirical associations identifiable in our sample between cultural and personal constructs as well as the indirect mediating effects that personal constructs might have on relations between cultural constructs and adolescent pregnancy outcomes. The second half of the chapter is devoted to a discussion of the structural and functional properties of the adolescent pregnancy system as a whole. These properties can be best understood in terms of internalizing–externalizing processes through which both individual and collective minds develop.

DIRECT ASSOCIATIONS AMONG CULTURAL AND PERSONAL CONSTRUCTS

Family Environments and Personal Representations

A first place to look for relations between cultural and personal constructs is in direct associations among family environments, internal working models proper, and quality of thought. Is it the case, as one might expect, that the kinds of family environments in which children grow up influence their construction of personal representations? Reciprocally, is it the case that women's intrapsychic, personal representations of themselves in relationships with others constrain the kinds of interpersonal relationships they can have with other people and thus the kinds of family environments they construct for their daughters?

Theoretically, the perspectives taken by LeVine (1982), Loewald (1980), attachment theorists (Bowlby, 1973; Bretherton, 1985; Main et al., 1985) and others implicate family environments in the development of personal representations through the impact of environments on the quality of social and emotional interactions between parents and children. This impact could come about directly through structural and extended-kin networking characteristics of families, such as the presence in the household of one or two parents or other adults who can fill parental roles or the presence of varying numbers of siblings, cousins, or unrelated children. The impact could also come about indirectly through the impact of these environmental factors on parents' functioning as parents. As LeVine (1982) pointed out, however, whether and how a given variation in family environment will make a difference in individual development is very difficult to predict, as there are many sources of variation among individuals besides environments that can play a part in development and that can impact how environments are responded to and integrated into personal representations. Thus, although we might expect moderate empirical associations between environments and individual development, attempts to understand these associations in any specific sense would be highly speculative.

Conversely, LeVine's (1982) work, as well as research by Blos (1962) and many others (Barglow, 1968; Bierman & Bierman, 1985; Buchholz & Gol, 1986; Cobliner, 1981; Hart & Hilton, 1988; Landy et al., 1983; Miller, 1986; Schamess, 1990) suggest that personal representations themselves constrain the kinds of family environments that individuals create for themselves. In this respect, both the thematic content and structural aspects of internal working models are relevant, the first in terms of what individuals want unconsciously from their interactions (i.e., emotional and material supplies, victory over mother for father's affections, or a mature relationship), and the second in terms of individuals' relative tendencies to externalize their quests for the satisfactions of these goals in the contexts of their relationships with primary attachment figures.

Our analyses for both mother and teen cohorts confirmed the expectation of an association between family environments and working models proper, but not between family enviroments and quality-of-thought

Table 8-1. Family Environment x Internal Working Models

	Internal Working Model Proper					
	Deprived		Competitive		Mature	
Mother Cohort						
Family environment						
Downward	11	(.85/2.25)	7	(.41/.21)	6	(.33/.32)
Traditional	2	(.06/.08)	21	(1.62/.1.10)	11	(.48/.79)
Upward	8	(.40/.30)	12	(.75/.43)	8	(.40/.47)
Teen Cohort						
Family environment						
Downward	18	(.86/.69)	9	(.30/.43)	12	(.44/.39)
Traditional	2	(.13/.08)	11	(1.83/.59)	4	(.30/.15)
Upward	6	(.24/.30)	10	(.48/.50)	15	(.93/.94)

Note. Entries are frequencies. Numbers in parentheses are odds of being in a given internal working model proper category given a family environment category and odds of being in a given family environment category given an internal working model proper category respectively.

classifications.[1] As seen in Table 8-1, deprived working models were most closely associated with downwardly mobile family environments, with the odds of being deprived given a downwardly mobile environment, and vice versa being higher than for other combinations. Similarly, competitive working models were most closely associated with traditional family environments in both cohorts. Mature working models were highly associated with upwardly mobile family environments, and vice versa, in the teen but not the mother cohort. In the latter, upwardly mobility was most highly associated with the competitive model, and the mature model was seen most often in the traditional family context. Inasmuch as upwardly mobile teens reported higher levels of emotional support from extended kin than upwardly mobile mothers (Table B-1, Appendix B), it is reasonable to speculate that the emotional climates in upwardly mobile teen and mother families differed and that climates in the teen upwardly mobile family environment favored the development of mature working models more so than in the mother upwardly mobile family.

---

[1] Relations among family environments, working models proper, and quality of thought were examined in 2 three-way loglinear (SPSS–HILOGLINEAR) analyses, one involving mothers and the other involving teens. For mothers, tests of partial associations indicated two significant two-way effects: Family Environments x Working Models Proper and Working Models Proper x Quality of Thought. For teens, identical results were obtained. Best fit models in both cases consisted of these two interactions, $L.R.^2(6) = 7.85$, $p = .25$, for mothers, and $L.R.^2(6) = 8.57$, $p = .20$, for teens.

Cultural Schemas and Personal Representations

Within mothers. A second place to look for direct associations between personal and cultural constructs is in the representational realm. Looking at this relation from the perspective of individual mothers, one could imagine a situation in which a mother was of two minds—one personal and the other cultural—developing along different tracks, existing side by side and functioning separately and independently of the other. For personal reasons, for example, a mother might be unconsciously reluctant to loosen the libidinized or aggressivized ties with her daughter as an external object, to create the kind of optimal interpersonal environment that could promote intrapsychic separation and individuation in herself and her daughter. Daughter's unwed adolescent pregnancy from this mother's personal perspective might be unconsciously welcomed. At the same time, this mother might have constructed a schema about the world in which she grew up and currently lives in which represented life goals and means of achieving them are antithetical to an adolescent pregnancy outcome for daughter. Whereas these two kinds of representations might conflict and create an internal experience of disequilibrium, one might say that they reflect separate but interacting lines of mental development.

In an alternative scenario, a person might also be of two minds, but these two minds would constitute two poles of the same representational unity. A mother's view of the world, of the necessities, the opportunities, the possibilities, and the means of achieving them, may reflect not only her life experiences growing up in nested environments but her personal, mostly unconscious view of herself in relationships with others. A woman who grows up with the unconscious view of herself as deprived in relationships with parents, for example, may unconsciously respond to other adults, peers, and representatives of social institutions in such a way that the experience of deprivation is re-created repeatedly. This woman's experience of her social world will be different from a mother who emerges from adolescence with a view of herself as an autonomous yet still connected being. From these different social experiences, these two women may construct different schemas of the possibilities and opportunities offered in society for work and for love and of the means available or required to achieve these goals.

Findings from our analyses examining relations among mothers' cultural schemas and mothers' and daughters' personal representations offered more support for the second than the first alternative.[2] Mothers'

---

[2] Two loglinear analyses (SPSS–HILOGLINEAR) were performed examining relations among mothers' cultural schemas and mothers' and daughters' personal representations. Personal representations in the first analysis were represented by the working model proper variable and in the second by the quality-of-thought variable.

cultural schemas, implied by their inconsistent or consistent attitudes and modes of communication toward daughters about adolescent sexuality, were directly associated with their internal working models. As in the example used in the previous paragraph, mothers with deprived models were less likely than other mothers to portray daughters as trustworthy and responsible for their own behavior without the need for tight restrictions or copious information about sex, pregnancy, and birth control (the consistent, nonrestrictive and noninformative schema). The percentages of consistent, nonrestrictive and noninformative schemas were 5% for deprived mothers versus 26% and 35% for competitive and mature mothers, respectively. Conversely, mothers with mature models were less likely than other mothers to portray daughters as in grave danger from boys lurking around every corner, while giving daughters minimal information about sex and pregnancy and warning against the use of birth control pills. Percentages of the inconsistent, restrictive but noninformative schema were 8% for mature mothers versus 24% and 33% for deprived and competitive mothers, respectively. These two extreme cells accounted for most of the variance in the relation between the two constructs.

Within dyads. Looking at the relation between cultural and personal representations from the perspective of the mother–daughter dyad, the consistency or inconsistency of mothers' communications to daughters are likely to be important aspects of the interactions between mothers and daughters from which daughters construct working models. We have already seen in chapter 6 how both mothers' and daughters' unconscious personal representations develop, are maintained, and are revised in a matrix to which both partners make continual, ongoing contributions. Mothers' cultural schemas, manifested in the consistency or inconsistency of communications about daughters' sexuality, may also enter into the mix from which daughters develop representations of their attachment relationships or from which they develop characteristic attentional/representational states of mind or qualities of thought in relation to these representations.

In the first analysis using the working model proper variable for both mothers and daughters, the best fit model included 2 two-way associations—one between mothers' cultural schemas and working models proper and the other between mothers' and daughters' working models proper, L.R.^{2}(18) = 21.99, p = 232. Partial chi-squares from tests of partial associations were χ^2(6, N = 174) = 15.17, p = .019, for the Mother Schema × Mother Working Model Proper association, and χ^2(6, N = 174) = 12.04, p = .017, for the Mother x Daughter Working Models Proper association.

In the second analysis using the quality-of-thought variable for mothers and daughters, the best fit model consisted of a two-way association between mothers' cultural schemas and daughters' quality of thought, L.R.^{2}(24) = 29.29, p = .209. The partial chi-square for this two-way association was χ^2(6, N = 174) = 16.30, p = .01.

Analyses of relations among mothers' cultural schemas and mothers' and daughters' personal representations revealed a relation between mothers' cultural schemas and daughters' qualities of thought, but not between the former and daughters' working models proper. The lambda statistic indicated that mothers' cultural schemas predicted daughters' quality of thought to a greater extent than the reverse (23% vs. 13% reduction of error). The pattern of relations between these two constructs indicated that daughters whose mothers were restrictive, whether inconsistent or consistent, most often exhibited the dismissing quality of thought (60% and 45% for daughters of inconsistent and consistent mothers, respectively). Daughters whose mothers were nonrestrictive were most often secure (43%) if mothers were informative, but preoccupied (60%) if mothers were uninformative.

That there would be a relationship between *how* daughters talk and relate to interviewers in the AAI situation (i.e., their quality of thought) and *how* mothers communicate with and to daughters is understandable from Main's (1995) perspective of quality of thought as an attentional/representational state. This state develops in the interactional matrix with mother and other important attachment figures and is transferred to the interviewer in the interview situation. The pattern of relations just described shows not a one-to-one correspondence between mothers' and daughters' modes, but rather an attempt by girls to distance themselves from mothers who are especially forceful in their restrictiveness and tend to interject or intrude themselves in daughters' lives, to continually access mothers who tend to give daughters more space and freedom to decide for themselves, or to open up to mothers who give information but do not attempt to control. Conversely, mothers' modes of communicating, which carry implicit meanings regarding their perspectives on daughters' adolescent sexuality, may also reflect mothers' side of the communication coin with daughters. That is, mothers with daughters who tend to dismiss them may work harder in the interaction to get their points across and thus come across as more restrictive than mothers whose daughters are preoccupied with their relationships or more open and flexible in receiving and interpreting information.

Other Relations Among Personal
And Cultural Representations

Although a theoretical case could be made for both, mothers' cultural schemas in this sample were related directly to neither their representations of daughters' attachment relationships nor daughters' representations of their own attachment relationships.[3]

INTERACTIONS AMONG CULTURAL CONSTRUCTS, PERSONAL REPRESENTATIONS, AND ADOLESCENT PREGNANCY

Personal Representations, Family Environments, and Adolescent Pregnancy

Family environments and pregnancy outcomes are not directly related in either the teen or mother cohorts, as analyses in chapter 5 demonstrated. Further, evidence from the same chapter indicated that mothers' cultural schemas are no more or less influential in promoting daughters' adolescent pregnancy outcomes in downwardly mobile, traditional, or upwardly mobile family environments. In other words, mothers' cultural schemas do their work for better or for worse with regard to daughters' pregnancy outcomes regardless of the family environments in which they were constructed or are currently played out.

Here, the question asked is, do family environments interact with working models proper in influencing mothers' or daughters' pregnancy outcomes? Is it the case that working models proper differ in their effects on pregnancy outcomes depending on the family environments in which women grow up? For example, is it more likely that a woman with a deprived working model will become an adolescent mother if she grows up in a downwardly mobile family environment than in an upwardly mobile environment?

Results from analyses of family environments, personal representations, and adolescent pregnancy variables[4] indicated that odds for pregnancy outcomes expected from girls' or mothers' internal working model

---

[3] A loglinear analysis including mother's cultural schema, mother's representations of daughters, and daughters' pregnancy status yielded two-way effects between both representational variables and pregnancy but not between the two representational variables.

[4] Two loglinear analyses were conducted for teens and two for mothers. For both cohorts, these analyses examined relations among (a) family environments, working models proper, and adolescent pregnancy outcomes and (b) family environments, quality-of-thought classifications, and pregnancy outcomes. For analyses involving working models proper, 2 two-way effects were retained in the final, preferred model: Family Environment x Working Models Proper, and Working Models Proper x Pregnancy Outcomes. Three-way

classifications are unchanged by the addition of the family environment variable in the equation. Like mothers' cultural schemas, daughters' working models proper do their work for better or for worse with respect to daughters' adolescent pregnancy outcomes regardless of the family environments in which daughters grow up. Thus, whereas family environments in our sample are contexts for the construction of working models and whereas working models strongly influence adolescent pregnancy outcomes, family environments and working models proper do not interact in the adolescent pregnancy equation.

Cultural Schemas, Personal Schemas, And Adolescent Pregnancy

The combined effects of mothers' cultural schemas and daughters' personal representations on daughters' pregnancy outcomes were implied by women who talked to me in the ethnographic phase of this study about their personal lives. In these narratives, daughters' responses to explicit and implicit cultural messages communicated by mothers and other socializing agents seemed to be partly a function of their representations of personal relationships with mothers and other socializing agents. Put differently, cultural messages were responded to in ways that seemed to serve specific intrapsychic relationship functions.

Aretha, for example, stated that she became pregnant to escape from the clutches of Martha, her vigilant and protective grandmother who raised her. In retrospect, it can be seen that Martha behaved and talked in a way that manifested an inconsistent, restrictive but noninformative cultural schema in which adolescent pregnancy was implicitly encouraged. Martha emphasized the necessity for strict rules prohibiting dating and other activities with boys, but she inconsistently enforced these rules and combined forceful accusations of sexual activity with passivity and neglect with regard to the giving of information about sex, pregnancy, and birth control. At a level of explicit communication, Aretha's more or less conscious decision to become pregnant contradicted Martha's stated wishes; at another level, Aretha's actions complied with the implicit message communicated through Martha's overall presentation encouraging Aretha's adolescent pregnancy. In communicating this implicit message, Martha both expressed her own implicit beliefs and acted as a conduit of important cultural knowledge. In acting in accordance with this implicit

interactions did not reach significance in test of partial association, and they were not retained in the final models. For analyses involving quality of thought, tests of partial association revealed no significant interactions.

message, Aretha continued tradition and added to an experiential base contributing to the development of her own culturally constituted schemas.

From Aretha's tales of her childhood and adolescent wishes, fears, joys, disappointments, resentments, and frustrations, however, a more personal narrative could be heard in which Aretha's responses to Martha's explicit and implicit messages take on additional meaning. Thinking back to her childhood, Aretha remembered feeling loved, protected, attended to, and encouraged by her grandmother Martha who was raising her, but angry and resentful toward her biological mother who had left her with Martha and "gone on about her life." What this meant was that her mother had found a man to live with, whom she married and with whom she had many children. Aretha was on good terms with her step-grandfather, but she could not help remembering the frequent drunken brawls that took place all her life between him and Martha. Time after time in our conversations, Aretha would come back to these memories, expressing angry and resentful feelings that Martha and her step-grandfather had abused, neglected, and abandoned her by subjecting her to these terrifying experiences, all the while making themselves unavailable to her. At the same time, Aretha remembered being drawn to these scenes, hiding under the bed or some other place where she could hear and see what was going on. It was at these times, Aretha recalled, that she fantasized being rescued by her father whom she had never seen, who would come by in his truck and take her away.

When Aretha reached puberty, her memories of Martha's attentiveness and grandmotherly concern took on a different quality of frustration that she was forced to "be under" Martha all the time. Thinking back, Aretha was incredulous that Martha went to such lengths to keep her from having any fun. On several occasions, Martha even dragged Aretha with her on trips out of town, ostensibly because she did not trust Aretha to stay home with her step-grandfather. Aretha was tremendously resentful that Martha had a man, her mother had a man, her sisters and half-sisters had men, all of her girlfriends had men, and all she had was Martha. It was in this context that Aretha as an unwed teenager voluntarily had sex in her father's house with a man who was the son of her mother's friend. Once the baby was born, Aretha married her boyfriend, settled down with him close to Martha's house, and refused to hand over her babies to Martha as Martha wanted, but she agreed to raise them jointly with Martha.

Aretha's personal narrative emphasized her childhood interests in her grandmother's, mother's, and sisters' relationships with men, in the contexts of her own felt lack of such relationships and her fantasies of having an exclusive relationship with a father she had never seen. These contrasts between what grandmother and mother had and what she did not have engendered feelings of anger and resentment and were associated in Aretha's mind with her successes in snaring and having sex with the son of her mother's best friend in her father's house. One might infer from this an unconscious wish to compete with grandmother and mother for men, particularly for a man who symbolically represented father. Aretha's actions subsequent to her pregnancy, moreover, suggest wishes not to destroy her relationship with a grandmother whom she loved, combined with a determination not to accede to grandmother's demands to give away her babies.

Aretha's representation of what Martha thought and felt with regard to her adolescent sexuality and pregnancy, we argue, played an important role in her unconscious choice of actions to accomplish her personal goals. In particular, Aretha's understanding at some level of consciousness that her sexuality was of intense importance to Martha, that Martha both wanted and did not want her to become pregnant as an adolescent, and that Martha wanted Aretha's babies to raise may have been decisive in Aretha's ultimate choice of action. Knowing at some level of her mind that Martha did not want her to become pregnant and have a baby, for example, may have given Aretha an opportunity to compete and achieve victory by choosing the opposite course. Conversely, knowing at another level that Martha did want her to become pregnant and have a baby may have given Aretha the courage to defy Martha's explicitly stated wishes that she not become pregnant.

The narratives of women like Aretha, therefore, illustrate that both culturally constituted and personal schemas are directly at work in motivating adolescent pregnancy and suggest that personal schemas may be implicated in the process by which cultural schemas become internalized as a daughter's own. The final question asked in this chapter pertains to the *nature* of the interaction between daughters' personal representations and mothers' cultural schemas in the adolescent pregnancy equation. Are these variables interacting in the sense that the effects of cultural schemas on pregnancy outcomes differ as a function of daughters' working model classifications, or are effects of cultural schemas uniform across working model classifications?

Our analyses of relations among mothers' cultural schemas, daughters' personal representations, and their adolescent pregnancy status indicated that mothers' inconsistent cultural schemas raised the likelihood of adolescent pregnancy for daughters regardless of daughters' internal working models proper, and mothers' consistent cultural schemas lowered the likelihood of daughter's adolescent pregnancy regardless of her working model proper classification. As seen in Table 8-2, the effects of these two variables on daughters' pregnancy outcomes, like the combined effects of mothers' representations of daughters' attachment relationships and

Table 8-2. Odds of Adolescent Pregnancy for Daughters in Teen
IWM-p x Mom Cultural Schema Categories (Top Section)
and Factors of Increase or Decrease of Odds in Relation to
Overall Odds for Teen's IWM-p (Bottom Section)

	Mom Schema				
	I-#1	I-#2	C-#1	C-#2	Combined
Teen IWM-p					
Deprived	6.76	6.53	2.90	1.20	4.20
Competitive	2.31	2.24	1.00	.42	1.30
Mature	.59	.57	.25	.11	.29
Teen IWM-p					
Deprived	+1.60	+1.55	-1.55	-3.50	
Competitive	+1.77	+1.72	-1.30	-3.09	
Mature	+2.03	+1.96	-1.16	-2.63	

Note. I-#1 = Inconsistent, Restrictive but Noninformative;
I-#2 = Inconsistent, Informative but Nonrestrictive;
C-#1 = Consistent, Restrictive and Informative;
C-#2 = Consistent, Nonrestrictive and Noninformative.

daughters' working models proper shown in chapter 6, Table 6-4, were multiplicative and compounding.[5]

The bottom half of Table 8-2 shows, however, that the factors by which mothers' inconsistent schemas *increased* the odds of daughters' pregnancies varied directly in relation to the developmental status of working models proper, with odds for mature daughters increasing more than for competitive, than for deprived. Conversely, an inverse relation can be seen between the factors by which consistent schemas decreased the odds of daughters' pregnancies and the developmental status of working models. Odds for daughters with deprived models decreased more than for daughters with competitive models, which in turn decreased more than for daughters with mature models. Decreases in pregnancy odds associated with consistent, nonrestrictive, and noninformative schemas, moreover, were relatively greater across all working model categories than the decreases or increases associated with other cultural schemas.

These results, therefore, support both forms of interaction just

---

[5] A loglinear analysis examined relations among mothers' culural schemas, daughters' internal working models proper, and daughters' pregnancy outcomes. Two significant two-way effects were included in the preferred model—Mothers' Schemas x Daughters' Pregnancy Outcomes and Daughters' Schemas x Daughters' Pregnancy Outcomes, L.R.^{2}(12) = 5.257, p = .949. Both of these effects have been described in previous analyses.

described. Although the directions of the effects of mothers' inconsistent or consistent cultural schemas on daughters' pregnancies were the same across working models categories, their magnitudes varied both as a function of the developmental status of daughters' internal working models proper and as a function of the quality of mothers' cultural schemas.

THE ADOLESCENT PREGNANCY SYSTEM ASSEMBLED

Adolescent Pregnancy Outcomes

The findings from the larger-sample interview phase of this study, as summarized in Figure 8-1, suggest that adolescent pregnancy outcomes for teens in this sample are strongly overdetermined; they are directly or indirectly linked to sociocultural and representational processes in both mothers' and daughters' worlds. Before reviewing the overall trends implied in the figure, however, it is important to reiterate that this picture of the adolescent pregnancy system characterizes our sample of all poor African American women from a particular region of the country where families have a particular history and a particular set of current limitations and opportunities for living and working. This picture would not characterize a sample including families across a broader range of the socioeconomic strata. In such a sample, we would expect both income levels and family environments to be more directly associated with pregnancy outcomes. Likewise, this picture might not characterize a sample from a different part of the country where family histories and current living and working conditions are different.

The findings from this study indicate that when variations in income levels, family environments, family histories, and current social conditions are restricted to a fairly narrow range, other factors typically ignored in studies of adolescent pregnancy come into focus as influential in differentiating women who do or do not become pregnant as teenagers.[6]

---

[6] A line joining two variables in Figure 8-1 is indicative of a two-way effect retained in at least one loglinear analysis described in chapters 5, 6, and 8. As discussed earlier, loglinear analyses examined relations among three variables at a time, and therefore it was hypothetically possible for the preferred model in any of these analyses to include a three-way effect. No three-way effects, however, were retained. This method of examining relations among three variables at a time rather than including all variables in one omnibus analysis was dictated by the need to maintain a certain minimum subject frequency to cell frequency ratio. Had a much larger sample been obtainable, it is possible that such an omnibus analysis would have yielded a different pattern of connections.

Figure 8-1. Associations Among Components of Adolescent Pregnancy
System

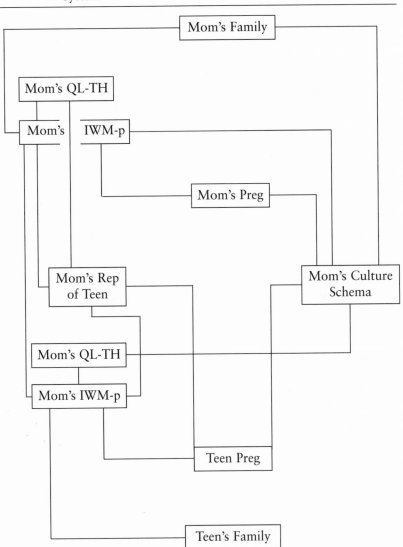

Considering the direct links to daughters' pregnancy outcomes in this sample, mothers appear as particularly potent forces. Mothers influence daughters' pregnancy status directly through implicit messages reflecting culturally constituted schemas of daughters' adolescent sexuality and through their personal representations of daughters' parental attachment relationships. Daughters' internal working models of their own attachment relationships also play a major and direct role in their pregnancy outcomes, as do mothers' working models in their own pregnancy outcomes. However, inasmuch as daughters' representations are joint constructions of mothers and daughters, mothers' hands in daughters' adolescent pregnancy outcomes are seen here as well. Mothers' and daughters' representations, as just described, have compounding, multiplicative effects on daughters' adolescent pregnancy status.

Considering the indirect links to adolescent pregnancy outcomes in both cohorts, family environments in both cohorts impact pregnancy outcomes through the mediating influences of personal and cultural mental representations. In the teen cohort, family environments are directly associated with internal working models proper, which in turn are associated with pregnancy outcomes. In the mother cohort, both internal working models proper and cultural schemas link family environments to pregnancy outcomes. Thus, in this sample of poor, rural African Americans, it is not family environments per se that account for the variance in adolescent pregnancy outcomes, but rather the mental representations of selves or of daughters in relationships or as sexual, childbearing women that women construct in family environments.

Personal and Cultural Constructs

Conversely, just as representations of mothers and daughters link adolescent pregnancy with family environments, so do family environments and adolescent pregnancy outcomes link mothers' personal and cultural representations to each other. Family environments and adolescent pregnancy experiences, we can assume, provide contexts both for the kinds of affect-laden interactions between parents and children that lead to internal working models and for the development of cultural schemas pertaining to adolescent sexuality and pregnancy. Personal schemas developing in family environments provide lenses through which experiences, information, and messages about adolescent sexuality coming from within and outside the family are received, interpreted, and acted on. Cultural schemas about adolescent sexuality formed in these environments reflect not just the information and beliefs communicated through cultural channels, but also individual women's personal ways of integrating and making sense of this information.

From the perspective of the internalization process described in chapter 7, family environments and adolescent pregnancy behavior patterns could be thought of as realms in which intrapsychic processes inherent in working models proper are externalized, given meaning in a specific sociocultural context, and then reinternalized with those specific meanings in the form of schemas about adolescent sexuality and pregnancy in this cultural milieu. Cultural schemas could be understood from this point of view as internal blendings of personal representations, actions and outcomes, and sociocultural meanings.

Generational Links

Generational links between mother and teen family environments and between mother and daughter adolescent pregnancy outcomes are also mediated by representational processes. Adolescent mothers do not necessarily beget adolescent mothers, and they do not necessarily create family environments for daughters reflecting those in which they grew up. Whether or not family environments are perpetuated appears from Figure 8-1 to be a function of the psychological characteristics (internal working models proper) of individuals making up those families, as well as of other factors (e.g., larger socioeconomic trends) not assessed in this study. Whether or not pregnancy outcomes are replicated across generations appears from Figure 1 to be a function of both personal and cultural representations constructed in family environments.

THE STRUCTURAL/FUNCTIONAL PROPERTIES OF THE ADOLESCENT PREGNANCY SYSTEM

In our conceptualization of the adolescent pregnancy system, therefore, there are three primary components: family-of-origin environments, personal and culturally constituted mental representations of selves and others in relationships and as childbearing women, and the adolescent pregnancy behavior pattern. Although not represented in our model, the system as so described is contained within a larger sociocultural context and has a history from which it cannot be meaningfully extracted.

The adolescent pregnancy behavior pattern in this conceptualization is viewed not as responsive to two separate although interacting sources of motivation (individual psychological needs and wishes, and sociocultural norms), both of which are conceived as separate and distinct from the behavior pattern itself, but as internal to the mental representational component of the system. Motivations for adolescent pregnancy reside in the minds of mothers and daughters who jointly construct personal and cultural meanings from their interactions together and with men. Development (or self-movement) in the system can be conceived as a process of working out, through internalizing–externalizing processes inherent in mental activity, tensions and conflicts between opposing forces. The onus for movement within the system, one could say (e.g., Bidell, 1988), is now placed on human agency.

This central integrating function of mental representations, and the dialectical processes of internalization–externalization that move the adolescent pregnancy system, are evident in the contexts of three bipolar relations that bind the system together: relations between mother and daughter, actions and representations, and culture and psyche.

With respect to the mother–daughter relation, the interpenetration of personal representations can be seen as the product of an internalizing–externalizing cycle. By externalizing the dynamics inherent in working models of themselves, their own relationships, or the others' relationships into the mother–daughter intrapsychic and interpersonal interactional matrices, both parties make contributions to these interactions which are then reinterpreted and reinternalized as components of continually developing working models. Inasmuch as mother and daughter working models develop together in the same interactional matrix through internalizing–externalizing processes, they partake of one another organically and are necessarily interrelated.

With respect to the action-representation relation, adolescent pregnancy behavior patterns can be conceived as enactments (representations through action) of mothers' and daughters' personal and cultural representations of selves and others in relationships. That is, women who have or have not become pregnant as adolescents have translated their own and their mothers' various personal and cultural mental representations into action. These "enactive representations," conversely, feed back into personal and cultural representations through their impact on both intrapsychic and interpersonal interactions. Enactments confirm, disconfirm, elaborate, or modify women's intrapsychic representations of selves in relationships with others and in mating and childbearing roles, and they shape the quality of interpersonal interactions with people in the larger, external sociocultural environment.

With respect to the culture–psyche relation, interpersonal family environments—beginning with the environment of the mother–infant matrix and extending ever outward to include parents, siblings, cousins, and other extended kin—are the immediate cultural contexts within which personal representations or working models are constructed. Into these environments, dynamics inherent in developing personal representations can be externalized or projected, shaped and defined, and then reinternalized in new shapes and forms. A further blending of culture and psyche takes place at the level of representations. Personal representations enter into the eventual construction of cultural schemas through the interpretations they lend on what is or is not possible or required for success in the present-day environment and on the meanings attributed by daughters to mothers' implicit and explicit messages about adolescent sexuality.

Conclusions

In this book, I re-posed some general questions of long-standing interest to psychologists and anthropolgists (e.g., D'Andrade, 1992; LeVine, 1982; Shweder & Sullivan, 1990; Strauss, 1992) about relations among culture, psyche, and behavior. These were: What motivates people in a given population or culture to put so much effort into doing some things rather than other things? How do people make the public information they are exposed to into their own thoughts and feelings? Put differently, what is the nature of the process by which frequently conflicting, inconsistent, and sometimes only implicit social messages become experienced by individuals as relatively coherent thoughts and feelings of their own? How is it that some cultural constructs acquire motivational force for some individuals in a culture but not others? Is it the case that no other forces besides culturally defined realities are required to explain why we do what we do?

The research described herein allows for some tentative answers to these questions as they apply to the specific case of adolescent pregnancy in the River Parish region of rural Louisiana.[1] Adolescent pregnancy in this population is well-suited for a study of relations among culture, psyche and behavior because it is and historically has been a frequently recurring (phenotypic), socially significant behavior pattern (LeVine, 1982). At

---

[1] As described in chapter 1, rates of births to unwed African American teenage girls on the whole have been moving within a fairly narrow but elevated range since at least the 1970s. Rates to unwed teenage girls in the White population, including those of Hispanic origins, have been dramatically increasing over that time period. To the extent that similar underlying factors are at work, what we have said and are about to say with regard to adolescent pregnancy in the River Parishes may be applicable in these other populations as well. Only further research can answer questions of generalizability.

the same time, however, not all women in this population of poor African Americans put so much effort into becoming unwed adolescent mothers. Although families of people studied in this research have lived for generations in conditions known to foster adolescent pregnancies (i.e., poverty, underemployment, racial oppression, and undereducation), there are still many girls who have not become teenage mothers. By contrasting those who have with those who have not, we are now better able to understand what motivates people who are all at high risk for adolescent pregnancy to action or inaction with regard to this behavior pattern and to understand the processes whereby environmental conditions conducive to pregnancies become associated with this outcome for some but not for others.

The Internalization of Cultural and Personal Meanings

The most important message to be taken from this work is that what motivates people in this community with respect to the adolescent pregnancy behavior pattern is not the environments per se, but how people interpret and understand at varying levels of their conscious and unconscious minds what environments and actions mean for themselves as individuals and as members of a social or cultural group. Environments, one might say, are where some of the action is; the rest is with individuals and groups of individuals who feel, experience, act in, and interpret environments. This message is important in understanding what keeps the adolescent pregnancy behavior pattern going in the present day, how it has evolved, and where it is heading. It is also important in devising interventions for reducing rates of teenage pregnancies.

Yet, although environments and individuals can be distinguished, they are not fully separate and distinct. When one looks across the spectrum of places where meanings are made, what is in one instance an individual or group of individuals making interpretations about the environment becomes an environment in the next instance to be experienced and interpreted by others. A mother, for example, is a maker of meanings in both her family and larger social environment and a psychological environment within which her daughter constructs meaning. Similarly, when one looks across the spectrum of generations, what is at the core of the meaning-making system in one generation (e.g., the meaning-making functions of the adolescent girl) becomes environment to be interpreted by her son or daughter in the next.

Moreover, communications from environments to individuals, including the explicit or implicit "public information" people are exposed to or the private unconscious or conscious messages delivered by parents to children, can be experienced by individuals as their own thoughts and feelings. The blurring and blending of individuals and environments is not just a question of point of view, but it is a developmental process whereby what takes first place on an external plane becomes reconstituted on an internal plane. Conversely, what is constituted on an internal plane can be expressed or enacted on an external plane where others participate in giving shape and definition to what is expressed or enacted.

This process, as I described in detail in chapter 6, is what theorists of varied disciplinary and theoretical persuasions have termed *internalization*. From the theoretical perspectives described in chapter 7, especially that of Hans Loewald (1980), both personal and cultural meanings are inherent in the mental representations that infants and mothers, children and adults, and adults and other social beings construct in interactions with one another. What is internalized in these interactions are the child's thoughts, actions, feelings, intentions, and meanings as responded to by mother in ways that strongly reflect her own unconscious views of herself in primary attachment relationships and of herself as a childbearing woman and member of her social group. What is externalized back into the infant–mother, child–adult mix are these same productions as interpreted and transformed by the child's mind. Inasmuch as representations of self in relationships and of self as a sexual being develop together in the same mind, they communicate with and inform one another. A developing girl's view of herself in relationships informs not only her own unconscious perspectives on adolescent pregnancy but also her interpretation of mother's. This individual— the teen girl become mother—with her own personal and cultural schemas, becomes and creates "environment" for her daughter. What develops from this process are both what attachment theorists term *working models* of selves in relationships and what cultural anthropologists and psychologists have termed *cultural schemas* of the demands and opportunities inherent in sociocultural environments.

Mothers, as the description of the internalization process implies, play critical roles in the construction of meanings and environments for adolescent pregnancy. One of the primary sources of variations in adolescent pregnancy outcomes is the capacity of mothers to be in empathic relationships with daughters that promote growth. Some but not all mothers are capable of sensitive, empathic readings of daughters' characteristics and potentialities, a capacity that reflects mothers' own psychological histories and represented relationships with primary attachment figures. Mothers whose own needs are primary and who have not achieved autonomy within themselves have a more difficult time allowing and encouraging the same within their daughters. Thus, for some daughters more than others, an unconscious sense of what mothers want with respect to adolescent pregnancy or other life issues and goals continues to play a major role in self-definitions and choices throughout life. A strong case could be made that, for these girls, what mothers want constitutes the primary determinant of what they want, regardless of whether daughters choose to comply with or oppose their unconscious perceptions of mothers' wants.

Fathers, although mostly in the background of descriptions in this book, also play critical roles in the process of constructing meanings. Fathers can help little girls through the intrapsychic processes of separation and individuation, primarily by providing an alternative attachment figure whom girls can love and turn to for protection from mother and with whom little girls can identify in their striving for separateness, competence, autonomy, and independence. What daughters and mothers want with respect to adolescent pregnancies and other matters is significantly influenced by their success or failure in negotiating this separation–individuation process.

Second, fathers' presence or absence in the household helps determine how families will go about obtaining what they need for economic and social survival. Families with two parents in the household generally have higher incomes and can afford to either consolidate resources within the nuclear family unit or construct kin exchange networks. Families with only mothers present, who have insufficient economic resources to consolidate or to share, are more often required to develop extra-kin networks in which multiple partners provide more advantages than single partners. Mothers' perceptions of what needs to be done for survival play a critical role in defining for mothers and daughters what is or is not desirable with regard to daughters' adolescent sexuality.

Third, mothers' valuations of relationships with fathers and fathers' valuations of their relationships with mothers, positive or not so positive, play a crucial role in what mothers want from their relationships with daughters, in what daughters want from mothers, and in the construction of daughters' and mothers' working models of themselves in relationships with men. Children without actual fathers present in their lives can and do have internal relationships with fathers that can function in ways similar to those constructed by children with fathers present. However, to the extent that having an actual father present facilitates separation/individuation and contributes to the valuing and appreciation of men and toward the formation of upwardly mobile nuclear families, actual fathers play a significant role in what girls in this community want and in the adolescent pregnancy behavior pattern.

The Historical Evolution of the Adolescent Pregnancy System

The message that the motivation for adolescent pregnancy comes from cultural and personal meanings constructed jointly by individuals and environments helps to clarify how the system has evolved and where it is likely to evolve in the future, given the absence of effective intervention. In the larger-sample interview phase, comparisons of three cohorts revealed that changes have occurred since the 1940s among poor[2] African American families in at least three components of the adolescent pregnancy system. Higher percentages of poor adolescent girls in the region of our study are growing up in downwardly mobile environments, are constructing deprived internal working models of selves in relationships with others, and are acting out their personal and cultural schemes in the form of pregnancies of unwed adolescents. Given what we know about the changes in the larger sociocultural–historical context during this time period and given what we know about the structural–functional properties of the adolescent pregnancy system, how can we understand these evolutionary developments? In what follows, one plausible scenario for these changes is described with the full awareness that others consistent with the findings of this and other studies are also plausible.

The scenario begins with the premise that family environments for African Americans in this rural community in the days before World War II were more homogeneous than they are today. The predominant traditional extended family was a viable structure given the possibilities of work for family members of most ages and both sexes, whereas political, economic, and social constraints limited the degree to which upwardly mobile families could facilitate transition of members to middle-class status. Traditional extended families in those days were more tightly organized and localized in the same geographical area, on the same plantation, in a row of houses on the same dirt road. Although some older women broke with tradition and sought education in nearby cities, the vast majority of African American women growing up on the plantations conformed to the typical pattern of working in the fields alongside mother from the age of 11 on, with time out for bearing and caring for children, getting married, growing vegetables, raising animals, and attending church on Sundays. In conjunction, the vast majority of men worked in the fields from sun-up to sun-down for $1 per day, 6 days a week (or 7, during grinding season). Education was minimal for most African Americans.

At the same time that family environments were more homogeneous, cultural and personal representations of individuals were variable as they are today. The expression in action of motivations inherent

---

[2] In describing these trends, we are referring to poor African American families living in this rural area of the South and not to the larger population of African Americans living in the River Parish region or elsewhere. The restriction of our sample to poor families does not allow us to draw inferences regarding the distributions of more affluent African Americans in this region among family environment, internal working model, or adolescent pregnancy categories.

in these representations was limited by the environmental forces we just described, but variability existed nonetheless. With respect to cultural schemas of adolescent sexuality, older women we talked to in the ethnographic phase, who were children or adolescents in the days prior to World War II, remembered how people reacted to adolescent pregancies back then. One older woman told us, for example, that in her day, if a girl became pregnant before marriage, she and her family would be disgraced and "driven out of town." Another older woman, when questioned about her own history of remaining unmarried for several years after the birth of her first child at age 15, stated that there was no problem with this because "everybody did it." Most older women we talked to, however, told us that becoming pregnant in their day as a teenager (around 18 or 19 or even younger) was unremarkable and becoming pregnant while unmarried was not particularly condoned but tolerated as long as marriage to someone followed shortly after. Although these women's memories of how things were a half century or more ago are no doubt infused with their current beliefs about adolescent sexuality and cannot be interpreted as veridical representations of past opinion, they do suggest the possibility that families and individuals in those days may have differed with respect to their implicit and explicit views about the desirability or acceptability of adolescent sexuality and pregnancies.

With respect to personal schemes of self in relationships with others, findings reported in chapter 6 suggest that in the cohort of poor women in our sample born in the 1940s and early 1950s, the majority constructed competitive working models, but a substantial percentage also constructed mature working models. A smaller percentage constructed deprived working models. Older women (and men) thus varied with respect to their representations of selves in relationships with others.

With the advent of the Great Depression and World War II, the structure of opportunities and demands emanating from the larger sociocultural environment of African Americans changed dramatically. Old ways of surviving slowly dried up, whereas new ways became increasingly open to African Americans in this and other parts of the country. Significantly, African American men and women in the region did not respond uniformly to this change in opportunities. Some started on the path toward upwardly mobility, others went toward downward mobility, and others tried to hold steady in their traditional family patterns. These different paths taken in uncertain times, we argue, are the products of human agency and likely reflect differences in what individuals brought with them to the task of choosing paths. Two things that individuals bring with them to any decision point are personal and cultural schemas representing hierarchies of goals and means for achieving them.

The existence of variability in cultural and personal schemas in the days prior to World War II implies that shifts in opportunities and demands were seen by individuals and families through different lenses, which in turn mediated differing responses to changes in the opportunity structure. For example, one might surmise that a girl who truly believes on all mental levels that she would be driven out of town for bearing a child out of wedlock, who is convinced that an unwed adolescent pregnancy is *not* desired or encouraged by her cultural milieu and representatives thereof, might feel a greater internal motivation than some other girls to choose a path excluding adolescent pregnancy as an intermediate step in the attainment of goals. Similarly, girls with more differentiated working models of themselves in relationships with mothers and fathers might be more likely than others to choose paths reflecting their inner autonomy and strivings for independence. Further, to the extent that more differentiated models imply a greater capacity for mature, heterosexual relationships, girls with these models may be more inclined toward and able to form and maintain upwardly mobile, nuclear family units made possible by new opportunities.

Those individuals who tried to hold on to what they had, and in particular to their extended-family support systems, were faced in these changing economic, social, and political post-War environments with a dilemma—whether to marry before or soon after childbirth or whether to decouple the birth of at least the first child from marriage. As the descriptive characteristics of traditional extended-family-of-origin environments in the mother cohort indicate (Table C-2, Appendix C), most households in those days were inhabited by a husband and wife, and most individuals were employed full time. These two characteristics go together in the sense that the availability of work provides sufficient resources to maintain a two-parent household, and a two-parent household is able to generate more resources than a one-parent household.

What changed progressively following the end of World War II was the availability of full-time or part-time jobs for men and women in this region, but especially for men. As times have changed, old ways of making a living in the region have steadily dried up at the same time that new and better prospects for employment elsewhere have not only improved but become increasingly visible and attainable. With the exception of an approximate 10-year period in which significant numbers of former farm workers were hired as unskilled or semiskilled workers in the petrochemical industry, the prospects of employment for poor African American men in this region have steadily worsened. The consequence is that young men and women who have abilities that could enable them to take advantage of employment opportunities elsewhere are faced with a choice: either leave the region in search of better wages or stay and make do economically in whatever ways possible. Those who for whatever reasons are less able to take advantage of opportunities elsewhere are chronically marginally employed or unemployed.

The aforementioned dilemmas of whether to marry and when have come into increasing focus as tensions have increased between possibilities of better employment in places far removed from extended families and continued loyalties to extended families and desires to stay close and share or give babies to mothers to raise. In days of old, the adolescent girl who became a mother continued living in the vicinity of her mother, father, and extended family regardless of whether she married before or after the pregnancy or not at all; the same held true for the father of her baby. Everybody, including the adolescent girl and her mate, regardless of their marital status, had an important role to play in the economic and social support functions of the extended family, roles that were contingent on the existence of jobs, however lowpaying. The prospects of a better life elsewhere were uncertain and dim. In this context, an adolescent girl could get married and have a baby, become pregnant and then get married before childbirth, or delay marriage for some months after her first childbirth and nothing much would change in terms of her economic prospects, those of her boyfriend or husband, or her proximity to her family of origin. In other words, the sociocultural and psychological functions of adolescent pregnancies could be served in any of these three marriage contexts.

In the present-day context, a marriage is likely to either take a young couple away from the region and their respective families of origin or bring together two people who have insufficient resources to support themselves, much less children. For men and women who are psychologically and otherwise prepared to take advantage of new employment opportunities, these opportunities and the income they may provide enhance the prospects of a stable marriage regardless of the age at which a woman might bear her first child. However, for other women who believe that maintaining networks, either extended kin or informal, are essential for survival and/or who are motivated internally to stay close to mother and share the raising of babies with her, these changed environmental circumstances make it less likely that marriage can be a viable arrangement. These women are reluctant to marry and move away from the extended family and mother and reluctant to commit to a long-term relationship with a man whose prospects for employment and steady income in the vicinity of her extended family are sporadic at best. Such relationships put an added burden on traditional extended family networks and, in circumstances in which kin networks are no longer viable, hamper the formation and maintenance of informal networks based on multiple sexual liaisons.

The impact that this dilemma has on marriage was especially evident in Martha's and Aretha's extended family. In this family, subtle pressures were brought to bear and felt by adolescents and young people of both sexes to stay close. Only Aretha and her husband were able to combine marriage with full participation in the extended family support and exchange network. Aretha's husband had grown up on the farm and was as assured as any laborer could be of continued employment there. Aretha's sisters and female cousins who had become pregnant as adolescents were married and living elsewhere, previously married and now separated from their husbands and living with parents, or unmarried and living without male partners in their parents' homes.

Whereas decoupling childbirth from marriage may have its advantages for achieving personal and networking goals for some women, the disadvantages are considerable for the psychological development of children. The association in this study between downwardly mobile families, which are characterized among other ways by the absence of two parents in a household, and deprived working models proper is consistent with this view. The point is not that children growing up in single-parent households cannot develop favorably or that the absence of two parents in a household is the only aspect of downwardly mobile families that predisposes children to the development of deprived working models. The point is, rather, that mothers in downwardly mobile environments lack the support of extended families, lack the emotional and economic support of a husband, lack sufficient and reliable resources for caring for themselves and for their children, and are likely themselves to have constructed deprived working models of their own attachment relationships. Fathers in these family environments are generally unavailable to children as objects of identification, as "representatives of reality" (Loewald, 1980, p. 12) who can help their children in the process of separation and individuation in their relationships with mother. In this kind of social and psychological environment, the difficulties for the mother–child dyad of negotiating a path toward psychological maturity are greatly increased. The consequences of failing to do so include among others the increased likelihood of adolescent pregnancy for children who become adolescents, greater difficulties forming and maintaining a stable relationship with a partner, and greater difficulties taking advantages of increased opportunities for social and economic advancement. These outcomes then feed back into the system and the downward spiral continues.

What I hoped to convey in this sketch of one possible scenario accounting for historical changes in the adolescent pregnancy system is that both external and internal forces are simultaneously at work in the process. This recounting of this scenario began by highlighting the dramatic shifts in social, economic, and political opportunities that have taken place for African Americans since the 1940s, for better and for worse. It would be a mistake, however, to leave the impression that changes in the adolescent pregnancy behavior pattern can be explained entirely by these shifts in the opportunity structure. How people in a community respond to external environmental conditions, circumstances and events—that is, the "kind of mind" (Loewald, 1980) that structures such opportunities—is as critical as the environmental conditions themselves in determining change. Ultimately, the most important determinants of change are the ways in which people interpret, utilize, transform, elaborate, and create external contexts. As Musick (1993) emphasized, the reluctance to acknowledge that people are the creators of their own desires, knowledge, and cultures, regardless of how poor they are or how politically sensitive this idea may be with regard to adolescent pregnancy in the African American population, is a serious impediment to understanding and to intervening in the system.

Implications for Interventions

Any thought or discussion of intervention must begin with an examination of whether there is a problem, and if so, how one should characterize the problem. Only after these questions are addressed can a decision be made about whether and how to intervene. In this specific instance, primary questions are, is adolescent pregnancy per se a problem? If so, how is it a problem and from whose perspective is it a problem? There is a second related but different question: Is adolescent pregnancy per se the problem to be addressed in any intervention? In other words, given that adolescent pregnancy *is* a problem, is it also a symptom of another problem toward which intervention efforts might be better directed?

With respect to the primary questions, the perspective taken here is that adolescent pregnancy in the present day *is* a problem from the perspectives of many people, including those populations most at risk for adolescent pregnancy, policymakers, society at large, and researchers who study the situation. Although there have been reports implying that adolescent pregnancy per se is not as much of a problem as has been commonly thought—for example, that adolescent mothers do not necessarily beget adolescent mothers (Furstenberg et al., 1990), that adolescent mothers do not necessarily end up poorer than their sisters who were not adolescent mothers (Geronimus & Korenman, 1991), and that problems thought to be associated with adolescent motherhood are considerably less for older than younger teen mothers (Brooks-Gunn & Furstenberg, 1986)—the commonly shared view with which we agree is that adolescent pregnancy per se *is* a problem in the present day and has become more of a problem for all concerned as a result of changes in both psychological and socioecological contexts.

With respect to the second question, although adolescent pregnancy per se is a problem in itself, it is still not *the* problem to be addressed in intervention efforts. Adolescent pregnancy is a behavioral solution that girls and the group as a whole have adopted to accomplish certain goals in the face of restrictions on what is and is not allowable in the family and in the society. It is a compromise between what is desired and what is felt as permissible, forged at a level of consciousness that is for the most part inaccessible to those doing the forging. It is a compromise that is all the more imperative and long-lasting because it is forged at this level of mind. The adolescent pregnancy behavior pattern can be thought of as *the* problem only in that the behavior itself feeds back into the forces that generate it and becomes a component of the cultural and personal representational schemas that are direct motivators of the pattern.

The "problem," as this last statement implies, is not only the adolescent pregnancy behavior pattern itself but the cultural and personal representational schemas in which adolescent pregnancies play an important role. The practice of adolescent pregnancy in the poor African American population will continue as long as people implicitly know the benefits and necessity of expanding and solidifying formal and informal kin networks, as long as mothers and other socializing agents unconsciously or implicitly believe that daughters' adolescent pregnancies will be instrumental in helping daughters to make their way in their current environment, and as long as adolescent pregnancy is an accepted mode of expressing and resolving conflicts inherent in mother–daughter relationships. Changing behavior patterns or external environments can support internal representational changes in individuals, but attempts to alter one without simultaneous attention to the others are likely to be unproductive.

This way of thinking has implications for whether and how to intervene in the adolescent pregnancy system. There is an argument to be made, after all, for not intervening, at least to any greater extent or in any different ways than have already been and are being tried. This argument might derive support from the declining rates of births to adolescent girls in the African American community over the last 5 years. If rates are declining, then we must be doing something right, and what needs to be done is more of the same until rates reach acceptable levels. This view that nothing or more of the same is the desirable course of action might also derive support from the perceived difficulty of the task at hand, that if cultural and personal internal representations are at the root of the problem, then the strategies that one might use to effect changes become much less clear and their prospects of success remote. Of course, the question in this case becomes whether a "stay the course" strategy is worth the risk that declining rates in the last years are *not* in fact indicative of an actual change in the slope of the trend line but are reflective of normal variability around an overall flat or even gradually increasing trend line that has been and is being little affected by current intervention strategies.

In our view, the trends identified in this research toward greater percentages of pregnancies of unwed adolescents occurring in downwardly mobile family and deprived psychological contexts in at least one poor African American population are sufficient reason to think seriously about and to be creative in designing interventions that can counter these trends. Whereas there are increasing numbers of African Americans in the population at large who *are* making the transition from poverty to middle-class status, the quality of life and the quality of mind for those who have remained poor have deteriorated, as Furstenberg et al. (1991) also noted in their study of present-day adolescent mothers as compared to previous generations of adolescent mothers.

Given the perspective that the problem resides first and foremost in the cultural and personal representational schemas of individuals, families, and communities, it is unlikely that interventions aimed exclusively at the adolescent pregnancy behavior pattern per se, or at external environments per se, will be successful. What I emphasize here is not that programs aimed at behaviors or external environments are misguided but that they are unlikely to have the desired effects on rates of adolescent pregnancies as long as more directly related internal phenomena are ignored. Interventions at these levels are necessary to provide contexts for representations to change but not sufficient to significantly alter rates of adolescent pregnancy because representations, to the degree that they are internalized and unconscious, are likely to be persistent unless focused on directly. The organic interrelatedness of these realms of human experience require a simultaneous assault in all realms.

Before ending with some general recommendations about directions for adolescent pregnancy interventions, I first mention three approaches that are widely discussed and promoted in the adolescent pregnancy literature and by policymakers, but that in the light of this research seem to have little chance for success unless combined with a simultaneous focus on internal dynamics.

First, it is unlikely that the pregnancy rate of poor, African American unwed adolescents will yield to straightforward educational measures touting the undesirability of adolescent pregnancy or the efficacy of birth control pills for preventing pregnancies. Women in this population know about birth control pills and know that the pill is effective in preventing pregnancy. In spite of this knowledge, mothers of adolescent girls in this study often actively discourage daughters from taking the pill, ostensibly because they believe that the pill causes physical or emotional problems. These beliefs are ways that mothers and others in the community have of explaining to themselves an internal, unconsciously motivated resistance to the notion of preventing pregnancies.

Second, the data from this study suggest that rising rates of adolescent pregnancies will not yield to reductions in governmental assistance programs.[3] The guiding principle behind this proposed solution is that poor teenage girls have babies in order to get or increase their Aid for Dependent Children (AFDC) payments. This, however, was clearly not the case in the families I came to know in the first phase of this study. Whereas some women were receiving AFDC payments, their primary sources of support were kin or informal networks of support and exchange. Proceeds from AFDC or other governmental assistance programs constitute only a portion of the resources that members of poor traditional and downwardly mobile families use to maintain networks of support and exchange. If this portion is decreased or eliminated, other existing sources will be relied on more heavily and new ones will be sought. As described earlier, other existing sources in rural Louisiana include decreasing numbers of full-time jobs; seasonal jobs; regular part-time jobs; irregular part-time jobs; illegal methods; and informal arrangements between men and women for procuring and sharing money, housing, food, and other resources that revolve around networks created and cemented by babies conceived and born out of wedlock to adolescent and older women. How willing individuals in these contexts would be to give up these informal arrangements and methods of procuring resources would depend in part on their perceptions of the real prospects for fulfilling economic and social needs through legitimate employment.

Third, whereas targeting poverty, schools, and jobs will be a critical component of any effective intervention, focusing on these components to the exclusion of less visible but nonetheless powerful motivators of adolescent pregnancy is likely to backfire. Adolescent pregnancy itself is a major impediment to improving the economic, educational, or vocational status of any population, and as long as this behavior pattern is being motivated by forces other than those in the economic, educational, or vocational domains, it will not only continue but remain as an obstacle to effective interventions in those domains. The "other forces" that motivate pregnancies, the personal and cultural representations and meanings, are deeply embedded in cultural and individual minds and will not easily yield to single-minded or even multifocused environmental interventions alone.

---

[3] Further evidence for this statement comes from a Rutgers University evaluation of the Family Cap program tried by the state of New Jersey (reported by David Liederman, Executive Director of the Child Welfare League of America, C-Span, January 2, 1997). Women receiving AFDC payments for one child born out of wedlock were denied increases in those payments for subsequent out-of-wedlock births. No change was observed in the incidence of out-of-wedlock births as a consequence of this new policy.

The findings of this research suggest some clear directions toward what we think will make a difference in adolescent pregnancy rates. In the realm of interventions in the external environments or socioecological contexts of development of families and individuals at risk for this behavior pattern, family environments in which husbands and wives value their relationships with each other and in which husbands (fathers) are consistently present and active in their children's lives seem to be especially important in supporting favorable psychological outcomes for children. That this would be a primary finding in a study focusing almost exclusively on mothers and daughters attests to the importance of men in the lives of mothers and children. In previous chapters I suggested reasons for this, including the economic and social support that a man can provide to a wife and children as well as the psychological benefits to mother and children of having a stable, good-quality relationship with someone other than each other. For both mother and child, fathers play an essential role in the outcome of the separation–individuation process. Although I hesitate to suggest specific ways in which good quality relationships between men and women in this or any population can be facilitated through intervention, perhaps one idea is to focus resources on the maintenance and support of naturally existing traditional extended families, in which stable marriages can be maintained in the face of relatively limited resources and which are stepping stones or transitional pathways to the upwardly mobile nuclear family form. How this might be done specifically is not within the scope of my imagination.

The clearest direction for intervention suggested by this research is that efforts must be targeted at the level of cultural and personal representations in which adolescent pregnancies, as we have seen, play important roles. Again, although I hesitate to suggest specific programs, two general approaches can be envisioned.

One approach would be aimed at helping mothers, fathers, grandparents, and children to externalize internal representations so that they can be reflected on and changed. Loewald (1980) and others (e.g., Fraiberg, Adelson, & Shapiro, 1975) suggested that there are times in a person's life when opportunities are ripe for psychological reorganization. Adolescence is one, pregnancies and childbearing are another, menopause may be another, as are critical points along the way in the process of separating and individuating in relationships with parents, children, and other attachment figures. The reason why these are critical times in a person's life is that internal conflicts are closer to the surface of a person's mind and are thus more readily externalized in conscious thought or even in communications with others. It is only by externalizing internalized conflicts inherent in representations that one can hope to modify internal representations through the effects of new experiences, contemplation, or interpretations and comments from self and others. Interventions with this goal, then, would be designed and constructed to facilitate, observe, talk about, and revise externalized internal representations.

Three reports of interventions with high-risk mothers and their infants conducted by "therapists" with varying levels of training illustrate this approach. Although all three examples given here include mothers and infants, one can envision similar kinds of interventions with any combination of family members at any ages.

Fraiberg et al. (1975), in an account of interventions with high-risk mothers and their failing to raise thriving babies, described how therapists' observations that in effect externalized in the conversational space between therapist and mother the internalized "ghosts" in these mothers' nurseries—that is, the pathological identifications that these mothers had made with their own mothers—led to an opportunity to think, feel, and talk about the ghosts, which in turn led to improved modes of relating between mothers and infants and subsequent improvements in their infants' developmental status.

A more recent application of this model in work with homeless adolescent mothers and their infants has been reported by Valliere (1995). Through weekly group discussions among adolescent mothers and a therapist with babies present, adolescent girls were helped to see connections between the ways they behaved, felt, and thought about their infants on the one hand and ways they remembered feeling in relationships with their own mothers and fathers on the other. Anecdotal evidence from this program suggests that in a relatively short time, some young mothers radically changed for the better the ways they related to their infants.

The third example of this approach—an intervention by Lieberman, Weston, and Pawl (1991) with "mostly Spanish-speaking immigrant mothers from Mexico and Central America whose infants were evaluated as insecure in the Strange Situation at 12 months of age"—was described in Belsky, Rosenberger, and Crnic (1995, p. 173). The focus of the intervention, which consisted of weekly 1½-hr home-based sessions over a period of 1 year, was to "respond to the affective experiences of the mother and child, both as reported by the mother and as observed through the mother–child interaction" (p. 174). By acknowledging and addressing the mother's own feelings and insecurities both in the present day and when she was a child, the intervenor helped her to then explore her feelings of anger and ambivalence toward others, including her spouse and her child. This intervention, which included an experimental and a control group, brought about changes in babies' free play and interactive behaviors with mothers after 6 months and changes in the quality of their attachment classifications after 1 year, which Lieberman et al. interpreted as manifesting an intermediate step in the ongoing reorganizations of infants' working models of attachment.

An alternative approach might be to focus interventions at the level of interactions between young mothers and their infants, with the goal of helping mothers to be more empathic with, responsive to, and sensitive with their babies to provide the kind of "sliding balance" that Loewald (1980) described as optimal in facilitating psychological development. Although we argue that mothers' behaviors with children are reflective of their representations and thus are one step removed from the most immediate "causes" of adolescent pregnancy, the relations among components in the adolescent pregnancy system illustrated in Figure 8-1, chapter 8 suggest that behaviors feed back into reprsentations and thus can have a modifying influence on them. One advantage of intervening at this level is that behaviors are observable and more accessible both to prospective intervenors and to those being intervened with.

In work with economically at-risk families in the Netherlands, Van den Boom (1990, 1995) reported success in modifying the observational skills and ministrations of mothers who had previously interacted insensitively with their infants—that is, both ignored their infants unless they exhibited high-intensity negative signs of distress and interfered with attempts at exploration. Changes in mothers' sensitivity were brought about in three home visits, in which feedback was provided to foster "contingent, consistent and appropriate responses to both positive and negative infant signals" (Van den Boom, p. 208). In relation to a control group, program mothers behaved more sensitively after three visits, and the quality of attachment exhibited by their infants 4 months after the program terminated was significantly more often classified as secure. The importance of this study is its demonstration that significant changes in relating between mothers and infants can be brought about through a relatively few interventions by therapists who are not necessarily highly trained.

Importantly, whatever intervention is tried, it is likely to work better if organized and implemented at the community level. Participants in intervention programs, those for whom services are provided, often do not see those services and the goals implied therein as relevant if imported into their lives by groups or individuals with whom they have no basis for identification. Whereas programs may be attended and services utilized, the meanings of these activities to those being intervened with are often very different from what the program developers have in mind. Many well-intentioned programs designed to facilitate parenting or other kinds of skills for adolescent mothers have foundered on the rocks of girls' perceptions that these programs are incidental or irrelevant to what their cultural reference group deems significant or important. Interventions need to be made through the auspices of community groups who are perceived by girls and their mothers as understanding them and what is required for survival and well-being in their own environments.

Finally, it is worth repeating that comprehensive intervention approaches are needed that target family environment, representational, and behavioral (action) components of the adolescent pregnancy system simultaneously. Without such approaches, modifications brought about through interventions in one component are likely to be counteracted by the many natural forces operating elsewhere in the system. It is for these reasons that the numerous worthy intervention projects focused on specific components of the system have had little effect on the natural evolution of the adolescent pregnancy system.

The Adult Attachment Interview (AAI): Coding and Derivation of Quality-of-Thought and Working Model Proper Classifications

A. THE AAI Q-SORT

In the Q-sort method of coding the AAI, one-sentence bipolar descriptors are rated on a scale from 1 to 9 according to their applicability to a given interview. For example, a quality-of-thought descriptor is "Provides only minimal responses (l.p.[1]—responds at length and provides unnecessary detail)." An interviewee who provided only minimal responses would receive a 9 on this item, where one who provided unnecessary detail would receive a 1, with interviewees falling somewhere between these two extremes receiving intermediate scores. On a content item such as "Is generally trusting in her relationships with men (l.p.—tends to view men as untrustworthy and unreliable)," an interviewee would receive a 9 if she described herself as trusting in relationships with men, a 1 if she described men as untrustworthy and unreliable, and an intermediate score if her descriptions of the trustworthiness of men fell somewhere between.

The quality-of-thought and content Q-sets used to code interviews in this study were modifications of Kobak's (1989) 100-item Adult Attachment Q-set, in which content and quality-of-thought items were combined. The 100 items in Kobak's (1989) AAI Q-Sort were originally derived from descriptions of interview transcripts used in the development of Main and Goldwyn's (1985) AAI classification system. The 100 items included 45 pertaining to organization (quality) of thought and 55 to the content of respondents' representations (working models) of their attachment relationships. In Kobak et al.'s (1989) research, classifications

---

[1] l.p. = low point.

derived from correlating individual respondents' Q-sorts with secure/insecure and deactivating/hyperactivating (dismissing/preoccupying) prototypes correlated highly with classifications derived from Main and Goldwyn's coding system.

In the larger-sample interview phase of this study, we wrote an additional 25 Q-sort items to supplement the 100 from Kobak's deck in order to reflect themes in our interviews not fully captured by his items. The final deck of 125 items was subsequently divided in two—one consisting of 45 quality-of-thought items and the other of 80 thematic content items. Each of the 261 interviews (mother–mother, teen, and mother–teen interviews for each of the 87 mother–daughter pairs) was sorted for both quality of thought and thematic content, making a total of 522 Q-sorts. Content and quality-of-thought sorts of the same interview were done by different coders (taken from a pool of 15 graduate and undergraduate students unfamiliar with the hypotheses of the study), and each sort of each type was performed by at least two coders (a third was used in the event of poor reliability). Reliability for content and quality-of-thought Q-sorts for mothers and teens using standard statistical measures was acceptable. Alpha reliability coefficients computed via the Spearman–Brown formula averaged .75 for quality of thought and .78 for content sorts. Quality-of-thought sorts for the mother–teen interview were unreliable and therefore not used in subsequent analyses.

B. Derivation of Quality-of-Thought and Internal Working Model Classifications

1. *Principal Components Analyses*

Two preliminary principal components factor analyses followed by varimax rotation were performed on the combined quality-of-thought and thematic content Q-sort items—one for the teen and the other for the mother–mother interview. The objective was to determine whether the resulting factors containing two or more items and with eigenvalues greater than 1.0 were homogeneous or heterogeneous with respect to quality of thought and thematic content. Of the 36 factors meeting these two criteria from the two analyses combined, only 2 contained both quality-of-thought and thematic content items. These two factors both contained only three items each and accounted for a very small proportion of the overall variance in the respective analyses. We can conclude, therefore, that quality of thought and thematic content are separate aspects of internal working models.

Exploratory principal components factor analyses (SPSS–X) followed by varimax rotation were then performed separately for quality-of-thought and thematic content items for the teen and mother–mother interviews and for thematic content items for the mother–teen interview. Factors were retained based on the Kaiser criterion (eigenvalue greater than or equal to 1.0), Cattell's scree test and interpretability. Scales were constructed from the pool of items correlating +/-.50 or higher with a given factor, and scores were computed for each scale by summing items with positive loadings and subtracting items with negative loadings.

2. Internal Consistency

The internal consistency of these scales was then examined using the SPSS–X Reliability program. Items that had the effect of reducing the overall internal consistency of a scale were eliminated. Scales meeting the minimum criterion of $\alpha = .80$ once these items were removed were retained for use in subsequent analyses. For both the quality-of-thought and internal working model analyses, factor structures were nearly identical for the mother–mother and teen interviews, indicating that these solutions have some generality across age groups in this population.

3. Scale Labels

For both teen and mother–mother quality-of-thought analyses, retained scales were labeled minimum quantity, expresses anger, and lack of insight. For the teen internal working model analysis, scales retained were Unavailable Mom, Available Dad, Mom Advice, Dad Advice, and Teen Felt Unique. For the mother–mother internal working model analysis, four scales were derived labeled Available Mom, Available Dad, Mom Advice, and Dad Advice. For the mother–teen internal working model analysis, three scales were derived, labeled Dad Available, Mom Gave No Advice, and Angry Dad.

4. Cluster Analyses

Scores for retained scales were entered into cluster analyses (Quick Cluster—SPSS–X), in which numbers of clusters specified corresponded to the numbers of categories identified for a given Interview x Q-Sort

Table A-1. Cluster Centroids for Mother Quality of Thought

Cluster	Minimum Quantity	Expresses Anger	Lack of Insight
1 Preoccupied[a]	-.30	.97	.33
2 Dismissing[b]	1.21	-.80	.88
3 Secure[c]	-.51	-.34	-.86

[a]$n = 30$. [b]$n = 22$. [c]$n = 35$.

Table A-2. Cluster Centroids for Teen Quality of Thought

Cluster	Minimum Quantity	Expresses Anger	Lack of Insight
1 Preoccupied[a]	-.03	1.00	.07
2 Dismissing[b]	.83	-.83	.78
3 Secure[c]	-.99	-.10	-1.04

[a]$n = 29$. [b]$n = 32$. [c]$n = 26$.

type in the qualitative analysis phase. Patterns were labeled according to the qualitatively constructed category to which they most closely corresponded.

a. Quality of thought.
Patterns of centroids resulting from cluster analyses of quality-of-thought scale scores for teens and for mothers were consistent with the qualitative characteristics of preoccupied, dismissing, and secure groups described in the attachment literature, and thus they were labeled accordingly.

Both preoccupied patterns (mothers' and teens') were distinguished by high scores on the Expresses Anger scale, with both groups producing moderate depth and quantity of information (the Minimum Quantity scale) and demonstrating a moderate degree of insight regarding relationship influences (the Lack of Insight scale). Patterns for both dismissing groups were characterized by minimal depth and quantity, low expressions of anger, and low insight. Patterns for both secure groups were characterized by moderate to high depth and quantity of information, moderate expressions of anger, and a high degree of insight.

b. Internal working models proper.
For internal working model cluster analyses of mother–mother interviews, six patterns of centroids emerged that were generally consistent with qualitative descriptions of categories.

Table A-3. Cluster Centroids for Mother Internal Working Model
Proper Variable

Category	Available Dad	Mom Advice	Available Mom	Dad Advice
Deprived				
Acknowledged[a]	-.80	-.57	-1.79	.05
Denied[b]	-1.09	-.90	.20	-1.61
Competitive				
Acknowledged[c]	1.20	-.64	-.66	.37
Denied[d]	-.48	.01	.58	.27
Mature identification				
Dad distant[e]	.51	.84	.58	-.72
Dad close[f]	.74	1.29	.68	1.13

[a]$n = 12.$ [b]$n = 10.$ [c]$n = 15.$ [d]$n = 25.$ [e]$n = 14.$ [f]$n = 11.$

Respondents labeled deprived (acknowledged or denied) had com-
paratively low scores across all scales, indicating a view of both parents
as unavailable and unhelpful in giving advice and promoting mature
behavior. A low but positive score for the deprived–denied group on the
Available Mom scale reflected these respondents' attempts to deny
deprived feelings with regard to their relationship with mother. A third
pattern portraying Dad as available and giving mature advice and Mom
as unavailable and failing to give mature advice was consistent with the
competitive acknowledged category, in which respondents describe themselves as Daddy's girl and mother as a hostile intruder in that relationship.
A fourth pattern, portraying a mother who is available but generally
unhelpful in promoting mature behavior or giving mature advice and a
father who is the converse of this description, was most consistent with
the attempts of competitive denied respondents to shift their loyalties from
a previously favored Dad to a previously unfavored Mom in the face of
Dad's rejection or abandonment. A fifth pattern, depicting Mom as both
available and giving mature advice together with Dad as available but not
giving advice, reflected respondents' mature identifications with Mom and
their view of Dad as around but not contributing much to their lives (the
mature, father-distant category). A sixth pattern depicting both parents
as both available and encouraging of mature behavior reflected a mature
identification with Mom and a valued relationship with father (the mature,
father-close category).

For the teen internal working model cluster analysis, the initial spec-
ification of six clusters yielded patterns that were uninterpretable. When
we increased the number requested to seven, however, five patterns

Table A-4. Cluster Centroids for Teen Internal Working Model

Category	Unavailable Mom	Available Dad	Dad Advice	Mom Advice	Teen Unique
Deprived					
Acknowledged[a]	1.93	-.50	-.57	-.76	-1.32
Denied[b]	-.50	-.43	-.92	-1.11	.74
Competitive[c]	-.09	.45	.27	-.07	-.37
Mature identification					
Dad distant[d]	-.44	-.80	-.28	.72	.24
Dad close[e]	-.51	1.19	1.29	.70	.76

[a]$n = 10$. [b]$n = 13$. [c]$n = 30$. [d]$n = 22$. [e]$n = 12$.

emerged corresponding generally to the two deprived categories, a single competitive category and the two mature identification categories, identified according to the same criteria as just described for the mother internal working model categories. In addition, two clusters composed of small numbers of respondents ($n = 4$ and $n = 1$, respectively) emerged that were most consistent with the competitive pattern, and were hence combined with the larger competitive group.

The mother–teen content cluster analysis, which generated the mother representation variable, grouped respondents into three main clusters and a fourth containing only two cases.

Patterns of centroids for two of the three main clusters corresponded to those expected for the Good Dad/Bad Mom and Good Mom/Good Dad categories derived from qualitative analyses. The third main cluster pattern appeared to be a combination of the Bad Mom/Bad Dad and Good Mom/Bad Dad categories—that is, Dad was represented as angry and unavailable, whereas the cluster centroid for the Mom Gives No Advice factor was close to 0. This cluster was thus labeled the Mixed Mom/Bad Dad category. The fourth cluster of four mothers was a clear representation of the Bad Mom/Bad Dad category. Because of the small sample size for this cluster, we combined it with the third cluster to form the Mixed Mom/Bad Dad group.

Table A-5. Cluster Centroids for Mother Representation of Daughter Categories

Category	Factor		
	Dad Advice	MomNoAdv	Angry Dad
Mixed Mom/Bad Dad[a]	−.72	.22	.48
Bad Mom/Good Dad[b]	1.19	.90	−.74
Good Mom/Good Dad[c]	.57	−.98	−.42

Note. MomNoAdv = Mom Gave No Advice.

[a]$n = 46$. [b]$n = lb$. [c]$n = 25$.

Coding and Derivation of Categories for Sociocultural Variables

A. FAMILY ENVIRONMENTS

1. Family environment information. In the larger-sample interview phase, information about the sociostructural and networking characteristics of family environments for respondents in the larger sample were gotten from mothers' and daughters' descriptions of the latter on the AAI and from the intake form. The AAI asks specific questions regarding where the respondent was born, where she lived, whether she moved around often, what her family did at various times for a living, whether she saw much of her grandparents when she was little, whether there were brothers and sisters living in the household or anybody else besides her parents, whether family members are living nearby now or whether they are scattered, and whether there are any other adults besides parents or grandparents with whom the respondent was close as a child. In addition, respondents spontaneously volunteered information about these matters in the context of their responses to other questions on the AAI. Intake questions pertained to the composition of the respondent's current household, ages, employment status, and financial contributions of family members.

Working in pairs, trained graduate and undergraduate students read each interview and consolidated information about respondents' family environment and extended-kin network on forms prepared by our research group. Coders completed the forms independently and then met to discuss responses and resolve discrepancies. Disagreements were arbitrated by a third coder. Mean percentage of agreement across items was .95.

From the demographic forms, nine variables were extracted—four reflecting structural aspects of the respondent's family of origin and five reflecting the extensiveness and viability of the respondent's extended-kin network. The four structural variables, rated on scales reflecting the degree of closeness to the prototypical nuclear family form, were mother's marital history, parent's employment history, head of household, and separation from birth parents.

Mother's marital history was coded on a 4-point scale from 1 (*never married*) to 2 (*married before or after first pregnancy/currently not married*) to 3 (*married after first pregnancy, currently married*) to 4 (*married before first pregnancy/currently married*). Parents' employment history was coded on a 3-point scale from 1 (*one or both parents on government assistance*) to 2 (*one or both parents employed part time*) to 3 (*one or both parents employed full time*). Head of household was coded on a 5-point scale from 1 (*one parent*) to 2 (*mother and boyfriend or other adult*) to 3 (*mother and grandmother*) to 4 (*mother and stepfather*) to 5 (*two parents*). Separation from birth parents was coded as 0 (*respondent was separated from birth parents during childhood or adolescence*) or 1 (*respondent was not separated from birth parents during childhood or adolescence*).

The five extended-kin variables were lived with grandparent or other kin, grandparent or other kin shared family residence, number of kin living in local vicinity, the number of exchanges of goods or services among kin, and the respondent's subjective feeling of emotional support from kin.

Lived with grandparent or other kin was coded as 0 (*no*) or 1 (*yes*). Grandparent or other kin shared family residence was coded as 0 or 1. The number of kin living in local vicinity was coded as (1 was less than 3; 2 was 3 or more). The number of exchanges of goods or services among kin was coded as (0, 1, 2 to 5, or more than 5). The respondent's subjective feeling of emotional support from kin was rated on a 5-point scale from 1 (*low*) to 5 (*high*).

2. *Component variables.* To search for patterns in family environment characteristics for the larger sample, we first constructed two composite variables—one, designated nuclear family, from the sum of four structural variables (mother's marital history, parents' employment history, head of household, and separation from birth parents), with higher scores on the composite variable representing a closer approximation to the prototypical nuclear family form and the other, designated extended kin, from the sum of scores on five extended-kin variables (lived with grandparent or other kin, shared family residence, the number of kin living in local vicinity, the number of exchanges of goods or services among kin, the respondent's subjective feeling of emotional support from kin), with higher scores on this variable representing a relatively extensive and well-functioning kin network.

Cluster analyses performed separately on mothers' and teens' scores on the nuclear family and extended-kin composite variables yielded four groups corresponding to two types of downwardly mobile families, traditional, and upwardly mobile. Patterns of cluster centroids for these types are shown in chapter 5.

B. Culturally Constituted Schemas

1. Component Variables

a. Communication styles derived from coding of joint interviews. Joint interviews were coded using the Analysis of Family Interview (AOFI; Nathanson et al., 1986), an instrument designed to rate videotaped interactions of family members. On 5-point rating scales, the AOFI rates eight dimensions of communication styles, two of which pertain to sibling interactions and hence are not relevant to our study. The remaining six are (a) clarity of communication (how well what is being said is understood by the rater and by the respondents themselves); (b) intrusiveness (the degree to which mother communicates "mind-reading" of the daughter by implying special knowledge about her or answering for her); (c) proportion of executive behavior (the proportion of total speech and nonverbal behavior of the mother of an organizational or managerial nature that attempts to regulate the daughter); (d) effectiveness of executive behavior (the extent to which parental executive activities are met with approval and implicit or explicit acceptance by the daughter and not by such responses as ignoring, laughing, continuance of offending behavior, disapproval, or contrary executive activity); (e) amount of conflict; and (f) resolution of conflict. Each videotape was scored by four students blind to the hypotheses of the study and who were trained to an acceptable criterion level of agreement with Mary Malik on pilot cases. Criterion level of agreement was $r = .90$. Using the Spearman–Brown formula to obtain composite scores, reliabilities in our pilot data were .67, .78, .82, .80, .89, and .83 for the six dimensions, respectively. The AOFI has face validity consistent with the concepts of Minuchin's structural family systems theory and Nathanson et al. (1986) demonstrated its usefulness in distinguishing relationship outcomes for pregnant teenagers with their boyfriends and families of origin.

Principal components analysis of scales from the AOFI using varimax rotation produced two factors with eigenvalues greater than 1, accounting for 63.5% and 16.9% of the variance, respectively. Scales loading on the first factor (labeled conflict) at .50 or higher were resolution of conflict (.93), amount of conflict (.88), and effectiveness of executive behavior (.75). This configuration suggests conflict between mother and daughter that is ultimately resolved by daughter's implicit or explicit acceptance of mother's executive activities. Loading on the second factor (labeled *mother's engagement*) were two scales that were virtually synonymous ($r = .86$): Mother's Intrusiveness (.92) and Proportion of Mother's Executive Behavior (.91). Extreme scores at either end of these two scales have negative connotations. Mothers who make very little attempt to regulate or to convey an understanding of what daughter is thinking or feeling would be termed, in Minuchin's (1974) theory, *disengaged*. Mothers who present themselves at the opposite extreme would be termed *enmeshed*, suggesting a failure to establish and respect adequate boundaries between the thoughts and feelings that are theirs and the thoughts and feelings that belong to daughters. Somewhere between these two extremes are mothers who are engaged with daughters in ways that do not negate daughters' initiatives and independence of mind. In Minuchin's theory, this attitude would be termed *flexible*.

b. Knowledge, attitudes, and beliefs about sex, pregnancy, and contraception. From the questions added near the end of the AAI, information regarding respondents' knowledge and attitudes with regard to sex, pregnancy, and contraception was consolidated on a sex and pregnancy form developed by our research group. Each form was completed by two students independently, who then met to discuss responses and resolve discrepancies. Information about the teens' knowledge and attitudes was derived from both the teen and the mother–teen interviews. If mothers and teens gave discrepant information regarding any item, the item was scored according to the account that was most credible. Each mother–daughter pair was rated on a 5-point scale for consistency of information about teens' knowledge and attitudes.

From the sex and pregnancy forms, we extracted the following information: (a) the sources of respondents' information about sex and pregnancy (family, friends, school or other); (b) mean number of sources of information about sex and pregnancy information; (c) the sources of respondents' information about birth control (family, friends, school, or other); (d) mean number of sources of information about birth control information; (e) whether or not the respondent used some form of birth control as a teenager; (f) if birth control was used, the person or agency from whom the respondent obtained birth control devices (mother, sibling, friend, health clinic, or other); (g) whether or not the respondent's mother put the respondent on birth control; (h) whether or not the respondent's mother approved of birth control; (i) whether or not the respondent's mother gave the respondent permission to date as a teenager; (j) whether or not the respondent dated as a teen; (k) whether or not the respondent was sexually active as a teen; (l) whether or not the respondent had a steady boyfriend as a teen; (m) the age at which respondent began menstruating; (n) mother's initial reaction to daughter's menstruation; (o) mother's attitude about daughter's activities with boys. Complete information regarding these items was available for 77 of the 87 dyads.

Thirteen items pertaining to (a) mothers' attitudes about daughters' menstruation, dating, boys, and birth control; (b) mothers' giving of information about sex, pregnancy, and birth control; (c) daughters' activities with respect to menstruation (age of first period), dating, and sexual activities; and (d) consistency of information given by mother and daughter were entered into principal components' analyses. Scores for two factors resulting from these analyses were incorporated as constituents of patterns representing mothers' cultural schemas of adolescent sexuality and pregnancy.

Dyads' scores on these 13 items, including one indicating frequencies of mother–daughter disagreements, were subjected to principal components analysis. Three components with eigenvalues greater than 1 emerged, accounting for 19%, 15%, and 12% of the variance, respectively. The first factor, labeled teen sexually active, included three variables relating to teen's actual sexual activity (teen has been sexually active (.79); teen has identified a boyfriend (.69); teen has used birth control (.60) and one describing teen's view of boys as not dangerous (.51). The second factor, labeled mother strict, consisted of items relating to mothers' attempts to restrict teen's dating and sexual activities (.78), giving permission to date (-.56), attitudes that boys are "dangerous" (.63), and mother's concern about daughter beginning to menstruate (.55). The third factor, labeled mother gives information, included items in which mother gave factual information about sex and pregnancy to daughter (.58), gave information about birth control (.82), and approved of or urged its use (.49); it also included items that reflected inconsistencies in the information given by mother and daughter (.58).

2. *Cluster Analyses*

Cluster analyses were performed on individuals' factor scores from analyses of joint-interview scores and sex, pregnancy, and contraception items. Resulting clusters representing the cultural schema variable are shown in Table B-1.

Table B-1. Cluster Centroids for Mother's Cultural Schema Variable

Cluster	Inform	Strict	Engagement	Conflict
1[a]	2.39	3.44	1.61	1.17
2[b]	3.21	1.83	1.80	3.26
3[c]	2.75	3.50	3.31	3.13
4[d]	1.41	1.53	3.65	1.82

[a]$n = 21$. [b]$n = 27$. [c]$n = 19$. [d]$n = 20$.

Analyses of Sociocultural Variables

A. Cohort Differences in Family Environments

Table C-1. Cohort Differences in Family Environments

Cohort	Family Type		
	Downward	Traditional	Upward
Mothers[a]	28	40	33
Older[b]	22	43	35
Young[c]	33	37	31
Teens[d]	45	20	36

Note. Entries are percentages of participant groups. One mother raised in an orphanage was excluded from this analysis. Chi-square tests comparing distributions of respondents between the three family types revealed significant differences between all mothers and teens, $\chi^2(2, N = 173) = 9.39, p < .01$; between older mothers and teens, $\chi^2(2, N = 124) = 9.16, p < .01$; and a marginally significant difference between younger mothers and teens, $\chi^2(2, N = 136) = 4.99, p < .10$.

[a]$n = 86$. [b]$n = 37$. [c]$n = 49$. [d]$n = 87$.

B. Descriptive Characteristics of Family Environments

Table C-2. Descriptive Characteristics of Downwardly Mobile, Traditional, and Upwardly Mobile Families in Mother and Teen Cohorts

	Mother			Teen		
	Down	Trad	Up	Down	Trad	Up
Nuclear family variables						
Head of household						
Mother only	63	3	14	44	0*ᵇ	13
Mom + other	25	6	7	27	29	0
Mom + dad	13	91	79	23	71	87
p^a		***			***	
Marital history						
Never married	42	0	4	49	12*	0
Divorced/Separated	25	6	4	41	29	6
Married/Postpregnancy	33	24	29	8	29	68
Married/Prepregnancy	0	71	63	3	29	26
p		***			***	
Employment status						
Govt. Asst.	89	0	7	59*	6*	6
Part time	13	3	4	41	41	26
Full time	0	97	89	0	53	68
p		***			***	
Separation from mom						
Yes (vs. No)	75	26	36	90	59*	23
p		***			***	
Extended-kin variables						
Participant lived with Ext Kin						
Yes (vs. No)	42	38	14	51	65	26
p		*			*	
Extended kin shared participant's family residence						
Yes (vs. No)	46	29	29	31	47	26
p		ns			ns	
No. of extended kin in close proximity						
> 3	67	88	61*	44	88	45
p		*			*	
No. of times received material goods from kin						
> 2	13	26	0	5	18	10
p		ns			ns	
Emotional support received from kin						
$\bar{x}^c$	3.5	4.1	2.7	3.5	4.3	3.4*
p		***			*	

Note. Entries are percentages of participants in family environment categories. Down = downwardly mobile; trad = traditional; up = upwardly mobile.
ᵃ Significance level for chi-square statistic comparing family environment categories within cohorts.
ᵇ Significance level of between cohort comparison for a given family environment category.
ᶜ Mean level on scale from 1 to 5.
*$p < .05$. **$p < .01$. ***$p < .001$.

C. RELATIONS AMONG SOCIOCULTURAL VARIABLES

1. Loglinear Analyses

Rather than performing a series of independent tests of associations among different combinations of sociocultural variables, we used a loglinear analysis to identify a model that best described the pattern of associations among sociocultural variables considered jointly. Loglinear analysis tests the relative applicabilities of various models of the observed frequencies in a contingency table, each specified by a given set of fitted marginal totals. The SPSS–HILOGLINEAR program accomplishes this by means of a backward search through hierarchically related models, beginning with the fully saturated model (those in which all possible marginal totals are fitted) and continuing until the best fit or preferred model is identified. The preferred model is one that cannot be simplified without a significant increase in the likelihood-ratio chi-square (L^2) and cannot be significantly improved upon by fitting additional effects (Brody, 1981). Once the preferred model is identified, the magnitude and direction of effects defining the model (i.e., its substantive meaning) can be estimated through the calculation of odds and odds ratios from the expected frequencies under the preferred model.

2. Relations Among Family Environment, Cultural Schema, and Adolescent Pregnancy Variables

To reduce the number of cells in the loglinear analysis of family environment, cultural schema and adolescent pregnancy variables, we first examined the table of partial associations indicating chi-square values and significance levels for main variables and interactions among variables. Variables appearing in any significant interaction with another variable were retained for inclusion in further analyses. Of the five sociocultural variables, all except the teen family environment variable were retained. Second, we inspected contingency tables showing relations between two variables at a time and collapsed across levels of variables displaying similar patterns of relationships. In this manner, we collapsed across the two "inconsistent" cultural schema categories and across the downwardly mobile and traditional family classifications. Variables (and levels) retained for the analysis, therefore, were mothers' family environment (2), mothers' pregnancy status (2), mothers' cultural schemas (3), and daughters' pregnancy status (2). For the loglinear analysis, we

Table C-3. Odds of Mothers' Cultural Schemas as a Function of Mothers' Family Environments and Adolescent Pregnancy Status

| | Mothers' Family Environment | | | |
| | Downward and Traditional | | Upward | |
Mother's Pregnancy	P	NP	P	NP
Mother's Schemas				
Inconsistent	3.13	1.38	1.00	0.00
Consistent (R/I)	.10	.36	.71	.25
Consistent (N/N)	.06	.11	.09	4.00

Note. R/I = restrictive and informative; N/N = Nonrestrictive and noniformative.
P = Pregnant as adolescent; NP = Not pregnant as adolescent.

specified a fully saturated model consisting of main effects and all possible interactions of these variables.

The preferred model selected by the SPSS–HILOGLINEAR program included a three-way association among mother's family environment, mothers' pregnancy status, and mother's schemas of adolescent sexuality, and a two-way association between the mother's schemas of adolescent sexually and daughter's pregnancy status. L^2 (9, N = 173) associated with this model was 6.58, p = .68. Table C-2 shows odds associated with the three-way association. Odds associated with the two-way association between cultural schemas and daughters' pregnancy status are shown in chapter 5, Table 5-2.

3. *Family Income and Educational Level of Mothers as a Function of Pregnancy Status and Sociocultural Variables*

Table C-4. Current Family Income and Mothers' Educational Levels

	Current Family Income		Years of Mom's Education	
Mom's pregnancy				
P	$10,179	(7,333)	10.55	(2.56)*
NP	$12,723	(7,810)	12.00	(2.98)
Teen's pregnancy				
P	$11,030	(7,988)	10.89	(2.66)
NP	$11,447	(7,239)	11.38	(2.97)
Mother's family				
Downward	$11,025	(7,858)	11.25	(1.77)
Traditional	$11,885	(8,090)	11.39	(2.87)
Upward	$10,794	(7,029)	10.68	(3.48)
Teen's family				
Downward	$7,649	(5,823)**	10.80	(2.62)
Traditional	$12,763	(7,946)	11.50	(3.32)
Upward	$14,899	(7,537)	11.31	(2.80)
Mom's schema				
Inconsistent	$10,449	(8,074)	8.83	(2.78)*
C-(R, I)	$11,705	(6,945)	7.19	(3.83)
C-(N, N)	$13,850	(7,792)	11.59	(2.41)

Note. Numbers are means (and standard deviations). *T*-tests (for two-level categories) and one-way analyses of variance (for three-level categories) were used to compare means.

P = Pregnant as adolescent; NP = Not pregnant as adolescent.

C-(R, I) = Consistent-(Restrictive *and* Informative).

C-(N, N) = Consistent-(Not restrictive; Not informative).

* $p < .05$. ** $p < .001$.

Analyses of Personal Representation Variables

A. Relations Between Pregnancy Status and Personal Representations

Table D-1 shows the odds of a mother or teen being pregnant or never-pregnant as a teenager as a function of her internal working model proper. Odds were derived from frequencies expected under the preferred models of relations among internal working model, quality-of-thought, and adolescent pregnancy variables. The preferred models were identified through hierarchical loglinear analysis (SPSS–HILOGLINEAR) and, for both mothers and teens, included 2 two-way effects: Internal Working Model Proper x Quality of Thought and Internal Working Model x Pregnancy Status.

Table D-1. Frequencies (and Odds) of Pregnant Mothers and Teens as a Function of Their Internal Working Models Proper

| Cohort | Internal Working Model Proper | | |
	Deprived	Competitive	Mature
Mothers			
Pregnant	16 (.45/3.20)	25 (.96/1.66)	10 (.24/.63)
Never pregnant	5 (.16/.31)	15 (.71/.60)	16 (.80/1.60)
Teens			
Pregnant	21 (.88/4.20)	17 (.60/1.30)	7 (.18/.29)
Never pregnant	5 (.14/.24)	13 (.45/.76)	24 (1.33/3.43)

Note. Numbers in parentheses are odds of being deprived, competitive, or mature given a pregnancy status and odds of being pregnant or never-pregnant given an internal working model classification respectively.

B. Relations Between Mothers' and Daughters' Working Models Proper

Figure D-1. Odds of Being a Deprived (D), Competitive (C), or Mature (M) Daughter Given Mother's Working Model Classification, and Vice Versa

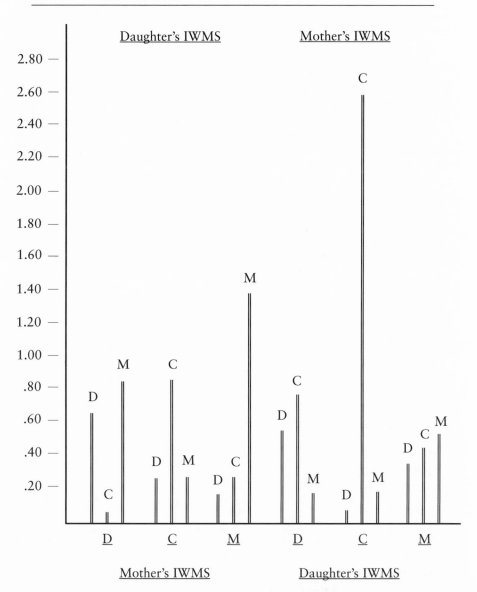

C. Relations Among Mother Representation, Mother Quality-of-Thought, and Mother Working Model Proper Classifications

Figure D-2. Odds of Mother Representation Classifications (Mixed Mom/Bad Dad, Bad Mom/Good Dad, and Good Mom/Good Dad) Given Mothers' Internal Working Models or Quality of Thought.

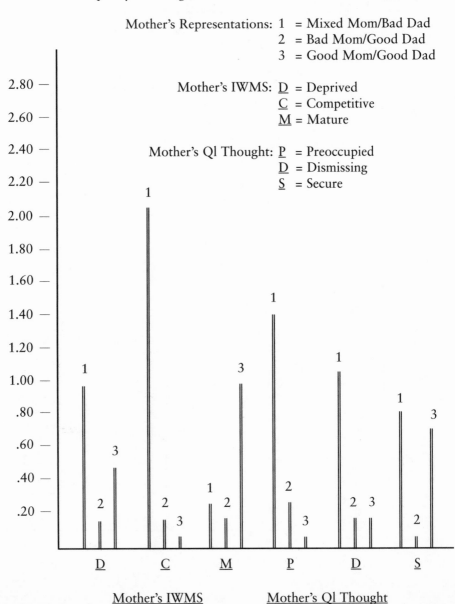

Mother's Representations: 1 = Mixed Mom/Bad Dad
2 = Bad Mom/Good Dad
3 = Good Mom/Good Dad

Mother's IWMS: D = Deprived
C = Competitive
M = Mature

Mother's Ql Thought: P = Preoccupied
D = Dismissing
S = Secure

Mother's IWMS   Mother's Ql Thought

D. Relations Between Working Model Proper and Quality-of-Thought Classifications

Table D-2. Cross-Classifications of Internal Working Models Proper with Quality of Thought for Mother and Teen Cohorts

Quality of Thought	Internal Working Model Proper					
	D_1	D_2	C_1	C_2	M_1	M_2
Mother cohort						
Preoccupied	8	7	6	7	1	1
Dismissing	1	1	6	6	4	4
Secure	2	2	3	12	8	8
Teen cohort	D_1	D_2		C	M_1	M_2
Preoccupied	8	5		5	10	2
Dismissing	1	8		14	4	4
Secure	1	3		11	5	6

Note. Entries are frequencies. D_1 = deprived acknowledged; D_2 = deprived denied; C_1 = competitive acknowledged; C_2 = competitive denied; C = competitive subcategories combined; M_1 = mature, father distant; M_2 = mature, father close.

Informed Consent Form

All persons who take part in this study are asked to sign a consent form. Signing this form means that you agree to take part in this study which is conducted by the psychology department at the University of New Orleans.

Both the mother and her daughter will be interviewed separately about their relationship and family history. These interviews will be audiotaped. Afterwards, the mother and daughter will be brought together for a brief discussion of topics brought up in the separate interviews. This discussion will be videotaped.

Please be assured that no information that you give us will be identified with you. All transcripts, audiotapes and videotapes will remain confidential and will be used solely for the purpose of research.

Signing the form means that you are participating in this study and understand what the project requires. Thank you for your participation. The above information has been explained to me, and I voluntarily take part in this study.

Signed: Witnessed: Date:

Signed: Witnessed: Date:

References

Ainsworth, M.D.S., Blehar, M.C., Waters, E. & Wall, S. (1978). *Patterns of attachment: A psychological study of the strange situation*. Hillsdale, NJ: Lawrence Erlbaum Associates, Inc.

Bakersmans-Kranenburg, J.J. & van Ilzendoorn, M.H. (1993). A psychometric study of the Adult Attachment Interview: Reliability and discriminant validity. *Developmental Psychology, 29,* 870–979.

Barglow, P. (1968). Some psychiatric aspects of illegitimate pregnancy in early adolescence. *American Journal of Orthopsychiatry, 38,* 672–687.

Bates, E., Benigni, L., Bretherton, I., Camaioni, L. & Volterra, V. (1979). *The emergence of symbols*. New York: Academic Press.

Belsky, J., Rosenberger, K. & Crnic, K. (1995). The origins of attachment security. In S. Goldberg, R. Muir & J. Kerr (Eds.), *Attachment theory: Social, developmental and clinical persectives* (pp. 153–183). Hillsdale, NJ: The Analytic Press.

Benoit, D. & Parker, K. (1994). Stability and transmission of attachment over three generations. *Child Development, 65,* 1444–1456.

Benoit, D., Vidovic, D. & Roman, J. (1991). *Transmission of attachment across three generations*. Paper presented at the biennial meeting of the Society for Research in Child Development, Seattle, WA.

Bernard, J. (1966). *Marriage and family among Negroes*. Englewood Cliffs, NJ: Prentice-Hall.

Bibring, G.L., Dwyer, T.F., Huntington, D.S. & Valenstein, A.F. (1961). A study of the psychological processes in pregnancy and of the earliest mother–child relationship: I. Some propositions and comments. *Psychoanalytic Study of the Child, 16,* 9–24.

Bidell, T. (1988). Vygotsky, Piaget and the dialectic of development. *Human Development, 31,* 329–348.

Bierman, B. & Bierman, J. (1985). Preoedipal fixation: its contribution to pregnancy in early adolescence. *Infant Mental Health Journal, 6*(1), 45–55.

Billingsley, A. (1968). *Black families in White America*. Englewood Cliffs, NJ: Prentice-Hall.

Blassingame, J. (1972). *The slave community.* New York: Oxford Press.

Block, J. (1978). *The Q-sort method in personality assessment and psychiatric research.* Palo Alto: Consulting Psychologists Press.

Blos, P. (1962). *On adolescence.* New York: The Free Press.

Blos, P. (1967). The second individuation process of adolescence. *Psychoanalytic Study of the Child, 22,* 162–186.

Bowlby, J. (1969). *Attachment and loss (Vol. I).* London: Hogarth Press.

Bowlby, J. (1973). *Attachment and loss (Vol. II).* New York: Basic Books.

Bowlby, J. (1980). *Attachment and loss (Vol. III).* New York: Basic Books.

Bretherton, I. (1984). *Symbolic play: The development of social understanding.* Orlando: Academic Press.

Bretherton, I. (1985). Attachment theory: Retrospect and prospect. *Monographs of the Society for Research in Child Development, 50*(1–2, Serial No. 209).

Bretherton, I. (1990). Open communication and internal working models: Their role in the development of attachment relationships. In R.A. Thompson (Ed.), *Socioemotional development* (pp. 57–115). Lincoln: University of Nebraska Press.

Bretherton, I. (1991). Pouring new wines in old bottles: The social self as internal working model. In M. Gunnar & L. A. Sroufe (Eds.), *Self processes and development* (Vol. 23, pp. 1–43). Hillsdale, NJ: Lawrence Erlbaum Associates, Inc.

Bretheron, I., Prentiss, C. & Ridgeway, D. (1990). Family relationships as represented in a story-completion task at thirty-seven and fifty-four months of age. In I. Bretherton & M.W. Watson (Eds.), *Children's perspectives on the family* (pp. 85–105). San Francisco: Jossey-Bass.

Bretherton, I. & Watson, M.W. (1990). *Children's perspectives on the family.* San Francisco: Jossey-Bass.

Brooks-Gunn, J. & Chase-Landale, L. (1991). Teenage childbearing: Effects on children. In R.M. Lerner, A.C. Peterson & J. Brooks-Gunn (Eds.), *Encyclopedia of adolescence* (pp. 103–106). New York: Garland.

Brooks-Gunn, J. & Furstenberg, F. (1986). The children of adolescent mothers: Physical, academic and psychological outcomes. *Developmental Review, 6,* 224–251.

Brown, S. (1985). Can low birth weight be prevented? *Family Planning Perspectives, 17*(3), 112–118.

Buchholz, E.S. & Gol, B. (1986). More than playing house: A developmental perspective on the strengths in teenage motherhood. *American Journal of Orthopsychiatry, 56*(3), 347–359.

Burton, L.M. (1993, April). *Multiple qualitative methods and models of intergenerational caregiving.* Paper presented at the Society for Research in Child Development, New Orleans, LA.

Burton, L.M. (1990). Teenage childbearing as an alternative life-course strategy in multigenerational families. *Human Nature, 1*(2), 123–143.

Children's Defense Fund (1986). *Adolescent pregnancy: Whose problem is it?* Washington, DC: Children's Defense Fund.

Children's Defense Fund (1988). *Teen pregnancy: An advocate's guide to the numbers.* Washington, DC: Children's Defense Fund's Adolescent Pregnancy Clearinghouse.

Cobliner, W.G. (1981). Prevention of adolescent pregnancy: A developmental perspective. *Birth Defects, 16*(3), 35–47.

Coen, S. (1992). *The misuse of persons.* Hillsdale, NJ: The Analytic Press.

Cohen, L. (1984). *Chinese in the post-Civil War South.* Baton Rouge: Louisiana University Press.

Compton, A. (1983). The current status of the psychoanalytic theory of instinctual drives. *Psychoanalytic Quarterly, 52,* 364–401.

Crowell, J. & Feldman, S.S. (1988). Mothers' internal models of relationships and children's behavioral developmental status: A study of mother-child interaction. *Child Development, 59,* 1273–1285.

D'Andrade, R. (1990). Some propositions about the relation between culture and human cognition. In J. Stigler, R.A. Shweder, & G. Herdt. (Eds.), *Cultural psychology: Essays on comparative human development* (pp. 65–130). New York: Cambridge University Press.

D'Andrade, R. (1992). Schemas and motivation. In R. D'Andrade & C. Strauss (Eds.), *Human motives and cultural models* (pp. 23–43). Cambridge, England: Cambridge University Press.

D'Andrade, R. (1993). Cognitive anthropology. In T. Schwartz, G.M. White & C. A. Lutz (Eds.), *New directions in psychological anthropology* (pp. 47–57). New York: Cambridge.

D'Andrade, R. & Strauss, C. (1992). *Human motives and cultural models.* Cambridge, England: Cambridge University Press.

Dean, A.L. (1994). Instinctual/affective forces in the internalization process: Contributions of Hans Loewald. *Human Development, 37,* 42–57.

Deutsche, H. (1944). *The psychology of women: A psychoanalytic interpretation (Vol. 1).* New York: Grune & Stratton.

Dougherty, M.C. (1978). *Becoming a woman in rural Black culture.* New York: Holt, Rinehart & Winston.

Dryfoos, J.G. (1990). *Adolescents at risk.* New York: Oxford.

Dunst, C.J., Vance, S.D. & Cooper, C.S. (1986). Teenage pregnancy: A prospective study of self-esteem and other sociodemographic factors. *Pediatrics, 72,* 632–635.

Ellwood, D. (1988). *Poor support.* New York: Basic Books.

Erikson, E. (1963). *Childhood and society.* New York: Norton.

Fogel, G.I. (1991). *The work of Hans Loewald: An introduction and commentary.* Northvale, NJ: Aronson.

Fonagy, P., Steele, H. & Steele, M. (1991). Maternal representations of attachment during pregnancy predict the organization of infant-mother attachment at one year of age. *Child Development, 62,* 891–905.

Fonagy, P., Steele, M., Moran, G., Steele, H. & Higgitt, A. (1993). Measuring the ghosts in the nursery: An empirical study of the relation between parents' mental representations of their childhood experiences and their infants' security of attachment. *Journal of the American Psychoanalytic Association, 41*(4), 957–991.

Foner, P. S. (1975). *History of Black Americans: From Africa to the emergence of the Cotton Kingdom.* Westport, CT: Greenwood.

Fox, R. (1967). *Kinship and marriage.* Baltimore: Penguin.

Fraiberg, S., Adelson, E. & Shapiro, V. (1975). Ghosts in the nursery: A psycho-analytic approach to impaired infant-mother relationships. *Journal of the American Academy of Child Psychiatry, 14*, 387–421.

Frazier, E. (1971). *The Negro family in the United States.* Chicago: University of Chicago Press.

Freud, S. (1915). Instincts and their vicissitudes. In J. Strachey (Ed.), *The standard edition of the complete psychological works of Sigmund Freud* (Vol. 14, pp. 105–141). London: The Hogarth Press and the Institute of Psychoanalysis.

Furstenberg, F., Brooks-Gunn, J. & Morgan, S.P. (1987). *Adolescent mothers in later life.* New York: Cambridge University Press.

Furstenberg, F., Levine, J. & Brooks-Gunn, J. (1990). The children of teenage mothers: Patterns of childbearing in two generations. *Family Planning Perspectives, 22*(2), 54–61.

George, C., Kaplan, N. & Main, M. (1985). *The attachment interview for adults.* Unpublished manuscript, University of California, Berkeley.

Geronimus, A. & Korenman, S. (1991). *The socioeconomic consequences of teen childbearing reconsidered* (Working Paper Series #3701). Cambridge, MA: National Bureau of Economic Research.

Grace, A.L. (1946). *The heart of the sugar bowl.* Baton Rouge, LA: Franklin Press.

Grice, H.P. (1975). Logic and conversation. In P. Cole & J.L. Moran (Eds.), *Syntax and semantics* (Vol. 3, pp. 41–58). New York: Academic Press.

Grossman, K., Fremmer-Bombik, E., Rudolph, J. & Grossman, K.E. (1988). Maternal attachment representations as related to patterns of infant-mother attachment and maternal care during the first year. In R.A. Hinde & J. Stevenson-Hinde (Eds.), *Relationships within families: Mutual influences* (pp. 241–260). Oxford, England: Clarendon.

Gutman, H.G. (1976). *The Black family in slavery and freedom.* New York: Pantheon.

Haft, W. & Slade, A. (1989). Affect attunement and maternal attachment: A pilot study. *Infant Mental Health Journal, 10*(3), 157–172.

Hall, G.M. (1992). The formation of Afro-Creole culture. In A.R. Hirsch & J. Logsdon (Eds.), *Creole New Orleans* (pp. 58–91). Baton Rouge, LA: The Louisiana State University Press.

Hamburg, B.A. (1986). Subsets of adolescent mothers: Developmental, biomedical, and psychosocial issues. In J. B. Lancaster & B.A. Hamburg (Eds.), *School-age pregnancy and parenthood* (pp. 115–147). New York: Aldine DeGruyter.

Harrison, A. O. (1988). Attitudes towards procreation among Black adults. In H.P. McAdoo (Ed.), *Black families* (pp. 215–226). Newbury Park, CA: Sage.

Hart, B. & Hilton, I. (1988). Dimensions of personality organization as predictors of teenage pregnancy. *Journal of Personality Assessment, 52*, 116–132.

Harwood, R.L. (1992). The influence of culturally derived values on Anglo and Puerto Rican mothers' perceptions of attachment behavior. *Child Development, 63*, 822–839.

Harwood, R.L., Miller, J. & Lucca-Irizarry, N. (1995). *Culture and attachment.* New York: Guilford.

Hayes, C.D. (Ed.). (1987). *Risking the future: Adolescent sexuality, pregnancy, and childbearing* (National Research Council), Washington, DC: National Academy Press.

Held, L. (1981). Self-esteem and social network of the young pregnant teenager. *Adolescence, 16*(64), 905–912.

Herskovits, M.J. (1958). *The myth of the Negro past.* Boston: Beacon.

Hofferth, S.L. & Hayes, C. D. (1987). *Risking the future: Adolescent sexuality, pregnancy and childbearing (Vol. 2).* Washington, DC: National Academy Press.

Hogan, D.P. (1978). The effects of demographic factors, family background, and early job achievement on age at marriage. *Demography, 15,* 161–165.

Jencks, C. et al. (1979). *Who gets ahead?* New York: Basic Books.

Johnson-Laird, P.N. (1983). *Mental models.* Cambridge, MA: Harvard University Press.

Jones, J. (1985). *Labor of love, labor of sorrow: Black women, work and the family from slavery to the present.* New York: Basic Books.

Kobak, R.R., Cole, H.E., Ferenz-Gillies, R. & Fleming, W.S. (1989). *A component process analysis of adolescent attachment patterns.* Unpublished manuscript, University of Delaware, Newark.

Kobak, R.R., Cole, H.E., Ferenz-Gillies, R., Fleming, W.S. & Gamble, W. (1993). Attachment and emotion regulation during mother–teen problem-solving: A control theory analysis. *Child Development, 64,* 231–245.

Kobak, R.R. & Sceery, A. (1988). Attachment in late adolescence: Working models, affect regulation, and representation of self and others. *Child Development, 59,* 135–146.

Koniak-Griffen, D. (1989). Psychosocial and clinical variables in pregnant adolescents. *Journal of Adolescent Health Care, 10,* 23–29.

Ladner, J.A. (1971). *Tomorrow's tomorrow: The Black woman.* New York: Doubleday.

Ladner, J.A. (1987). Black teenage pregnancy: a challenge for educators. *Journal of Negro Education, 56*(1), 53–63.

Lancaster, B. & Hamburg, B. (Eds.). (1986). *School age pregnancy and parenthood.* New York: deGruyter.

Landy, S., Schubert, J., Cleland, J., Clark, C. & Montgomery, J. (1983). Teenage pregnancy: Family syndrome. *Adolescence, 18*(71), 679–694.

LeVine, R.A. (1982). *Culture, behavior and personality.* Chicago: Aldine.

Lieberman, A.F., Weston, D.R. & Pawl, J.H. (1991). Preventive intervention and outcome with anxiously attached dyads. *Child Development, 62,* 199–209.

Liederman, D. (1997, January 2). *C-Span.* Washington Journal, Connie Brod (Producer), Washington, DC.

Loewald, H. (1978). *Psychoanalysis and the history of the individual.* New Haven, CT: Yale University Press.

Loewald, H. (1980). *Papers on psychoanalysis.* New Haven, CT: Yale University Press.

Loewald, H. (1988). *Sublimation: Inquiries into theoretical psychoanalysis.* New Haven, CT: Yale University Press.

MacLeod, J. (1987). *Ain't no making it: Leveled aspirations in a low-income neighborhood.* Boulder, CO: Westview Press.

Main, M. (1995). Recent studies in attachment: Overview, with selected implications for clinical work. In S. Goldberg, R. Muir & J. Kerr (Eds.), *Attachment theory: Social, developmental and clinical perspectives* (pp. 407–474). Hillsdale, NJ: The Analytic Press.

Main, M. & Goldwyn, R. (1985). *Adult attachment classification system.* Unpublished manuscript, University of California, Berkeley.

Main, M. & Goldwyn, R. (in press). Adult attachment scoring and classification system. In M. Main (Ed.), *Systems for assessing attachment organization through discourse, behavior and drawings* (working title). Cambridge, England: Cambridge University Press.

Main, M. & Hesse, E. (1990). Parents' unresolved traumatic experiences are related to infant disorganized attachment status: Is frightened and/or frightening parental behavior the linking mechanism? In M. Greenberg, D. Ciccheti & E.M. Cummings (Eds.), *Attachment during the preschool years: Theory, research and intervention* (pp. 161–182). Chicago: University of Chicago Press.

Main, M., Kaplan, K. & Cassidy, J. (1985). Security in infancy and childhood: A move to the level of representation. *Monographs of the Society for Research in Child Development, 50,* (1–2, Serial No. 209).

Main, M. & Soloman, J. (1986). Discovery of a new insecure-disorganized/disoriented attachment pattern. In T.B. Brazelton & M. Yogman (Eds.), *Affective development in infancy* (pp. 95–124). Norwood, NJ: Ablex.

Mbiti, J.S. (1969). *African religions and philosophy.* New York: Praeger.

McAdoo, H.P. (Ed.). (1988a). *Black families* (2nd ed.). Newbury Park, CA: Sage.

McAdoo, H.P. (1988b). Transgenerational patterns of upward mobility in African-American families. In H.P. McAdoo (Ed.), *Black families* (2nd ed., pp. 148–169). Newbury Park, CA: Sage.

Meier, A. & Rudwick, E. (1976). *From plantation to ghetto.* New York: Pantheon.

Meyerowitz, J.H. & Malev, J.S. (1973). Pubescent attitudinal correlates antecedent of adolescent illegitimate pregnancy. *Journal of Youth and Adolescence, 2,* 251–258.

Miller, B.C., Cristensen, R.B. & Olson, T.D. (1978). Adolescent self-esteem in relation to sexual attitudes and behavior. *Youth and Society, 19*(1), 93–111.

Miller, N. (1986). Unplanned adolescent pregnancy and the transitional object. *Child and Adolescent Social Work, 3*(2), 77–86.

Minuchin, S. (1974). *Families and family therapy.* Cambridge: Harvard University Press.

Moynihan, D.P. (1965). *The Negro family: The case for national action.* (Office of Planning and Research) Washington, DC: U.S. Government Printing Office.

Moynihan, D.P. (1997, January 28). The big lie. *Washington Post,* p. A-13.

Musick, J.S. (1993). *Young, poor and pregnant.* New Haven, CT: Yale University Press.

Nathanson, C.A. (1991). *Dangerous passage.* Philadelphia: Temple University Press.

Nathanson, M., Baird, A. & Jemail, J. (1986). Family functioning and the adolescent mother: A systems approach. *Adolescence, 21*(84), 827–841.

National Center for Health Statistics (1991). *Monthly vital statistics report, 40*(8).

Nelson, K. (1983). The derivation of concepts and categories from event representations. In E.K. Scholnick (Ed.), *New trends in conceptual representation: Challenges to Piaget's theory?* (pp. 131–151). Hillsdale, NJ: Lawrence Erlbaum Associates, Inc.

Nelson, K. (1986). *Event knowledge: Structure and function in development.* Hillsdale, NJ: Lawrence Erlbaum Associates, Inc.

Nobles, R. (1974). African root and American fruit: The Black family. *Journal of Social and Behavioral Sciences, 20,* 52–64.

Ogbu, J. U. (1981). Origins of human experience: A cultural-ecological perspective. *Child Development, 52,* 413–429.

Ornstein, A. & Ornstein, P. (1985). Parenting as a function of the adult self: A psychoanalytic developmental perspective. In E.J. Anthony & G. Pollack (Eds.), *Parental influences in health and disease* (pp. 135–167). Boston: Little, Brown.

Osofsky, J., Hann, D. & Peebles, C. (1993). Adolescent parenthood: Risks and opportunities for mothers and infants. In C. Zeanah (Ed.), *Handbook of infant mental health* (pp. 106–120). New York: Guilford.

Osofsky, J.D., Osofsky, H.J. & Diamond, M.O. (1988). The transition to parenthood: Special tasks and risk factors for adolescent mothers. In G.Y. Michaels & W. A. Goldberg (Eds.), *The transition to parenthood* (pp. 209–234). New York: Cambridge University Press.

Pattern, M.A. (1981). Self concept and self esteem factors in adolescent pregnancy. *Adolescence, 16*(64), 765–777.

Phipps-Yonas, S. (1980). Teenage pregnancy and motherhood: A review of the literature. *American Journal of Orthopsychiatry, 50*(3), 403–431.

Piaget, J. (1924). The language and thought of the child. London: Routledge & Kegan Paul.

Piaget, J. (1952). *Origins of intelligence.* New York: Basic Books.

Piaget, J. & Inhelder, B. (1948). The child's conception of space. London: Routledge & Kegan Paul.

Ploski, H.A. & Williams, J. (Eds.). (1989). *The Negro almanac: A reference work on the Afro-American* (5th ed.). New York: Gale Research.

Polit, D.F. (1986). *Comprehensive programs for pregnant and parenting teenagers.* Saratoga Springs, NY: Humananalysis.

Polit, D.F. (1989). Effects of a comprehensive program for teenage parents: Five years after Project Redirection. *Family Planning Perspectives, 21*(4), 164–187.

Polit, D.F. & White, C. (1988). *The lives of disadvantaged mothers: The five-year follow-up of the Project Redirection sample.* Saratoga Springs, NY: Humananalysis.

Radojevic, M. (1992, May). *Predicting quality of infant attachment to father at 15 months from prenatal paternal representations of attachment: An Australian contribution.* Paper presented at the 25th International Congress of Psychology, Brussels.

Rainwater, L. & Yancey, W.L. (1967). *The Moynihan report and the politics of controversy.* Cambridge, MA: MIT Press.

Ralph, N., Lochman, J. & Thomas, T. (1984). Psychosocial characteristics of pregnant and nulliparous adolescents. *Adolescence, 19*(74), 283–294.

Rice, K.G. (1991). Attachment in adolescence: A narrative and meta-analytic review. *Journal of Youth and Adolescence, 19*(5), 511–538.

Rosenberg, H.M., Ventura, S.J., Maurer, J.D., Heuser, R.L. & Freedman, M. (1996). Births and deaths: United States, 1995. *Monthly Vital Statistics Report,* National Center for Health Statistics, *45*(3), Supplement 2.

Sagi, A., Van Ilzendoorn, M.H., Scharf, M., Koren-Karie, N., Joels, T. & Mayseless, O. (1994). Stability and discriminant validity of the Adult Attachment Interview: A psychometric study in young Israeli adults. *Developmental Psychology, 30,* 771–777.

Sandler, J. & Rosenblatt, B. (1962). The concept of the representational world. *Psychoanalytic Study of the Child, 17,* 128–145.

Schamess, G. (1990). Toward an understanding of the etiology and treatment of psychological dysfunction among single teenage mothers: Part II. *Smith College Studies in Social Work, 60*(3), 244–262.

Schank, R.C. (1982). *Dynamic memory: A theory of reminding and learning in computers and people.* Cambridge, MA: Cambridge University Press.

Schank, R.C. & Abelson, R.P. (1977). *Scripts, plans, goals and understanding.* Hillsdale, NJ: Lawrence Erlbaum Associates, Inc.

Schwartz, T., White, G.M. & Lutz, C.A. (1993). *New directions in psychological anthropology.* New York: Cambridge University Press.

Segal, S.M. & DuCette, J. (1973). Locus of control and premarital high school pregnancy. *Psychological Reports, 33,* 887–890.

Shweder, R. A. & Sullivan, M.A. (1990). The semiotic subject of cultural psychology. In L. Pervin (Ed.), *Handbook of personality* (pp. 399–413). New York: Guilford.

Social Security Bulletin (1989). *Social security in review: The 1989 federal poverty income guidelines, 52*(3), 30.

Sowell, T. (1981). *Ethnic America: A history.* New York: Basic Books.

Sperber, D. (1985). Anthropology and psychology: Towards an epidemiology of Representations. *Man, 20*(1), 73–87.

Spiro, M. (1961). Social systems, personality and functional analysis. In B. Kaplan (Ed.), *Studying personality cross-culturally* (pp. 93–129). Evanston, IL: Row, Peterson.

Spruiell, V. (1989). On blaming: An entry to the theory of values. *Psychoanalytic Study of the Child, 44,* 241–267.

SPSS, Inc. (1988). *SPSS-X user's guide* (3rd ed.). Chicago.

Sroufe, L.A. (1993). Relationships, self and individual adaptation. In A.J. Sameroff & R. N. Emde (Eds.), *Relationships and disturbances in early childhood: A developmental approach.* New York: Basic Books.

Sroufe, L.A. & Waters, E., (1977). Attachment as an organizational construct. *Child Development, 49,* 1184–1199.

Stack, C.B. (1974). *All our kin.* New York: Harper & Row.

Stack, C.B. (1996). *Call to home.* New York: Basic Books.

Staples, R. (1988). An overview of race and marital status. In H. McAdoo (Ed.), *Black families* (pp. 187–190). Newbury Park, CA: Sage.

Staples, R. & Johnson, L.B. (1993). *Black families at the crossroads: Challenges and prospects.* San Francisco: Jossey-Bass.

Statistical Abstract of Louisiana (1990). University of New Orleans.

Stern, D. (1985). *The interpersonal world of the infant.* New York: Basic Books.

Strauss, C. (1992). Models and motives. In R.A. D'Andrade & C. Strauss (Eds.), *Human motives and cultural models* (pp. 1–20). Cambridge, England: Cambridge University Press.

Sudarkasa, N. (1988). Interpreting the African heritage in Afro-American family organizations. In H.P. McAdoo (Ed.), *Black families* (2nd ed., pp. 27–44). Newbury Park, CA: Sage.

Valliere, J. S. (1995). Infant mental health: A consultation and treatment team for at risk infants and toddlers. *Infants and Young Children, 6*(3), 46–53.

Van den Boom, D. (1990). Preventive intervention and the quality of mother–infant interaction and infant exploration in irritable infants. In W. Koops et al. (Eds.), *Developmental psychology behind the dikes* (pp. 249–270). Amsterdam: Eburon.

Van den Boom, D. (1995). The influence of temperament and mothering on attachment and exploration. *Child Development, 50,* (Nos. 1–2), 41–65.

Van Ilzendoorn, M.H. (1995). Adult attachment representations, parental responsiveness and infant attachment: A meta-analysis on the predictive validity of the Adult Attachment Interview. *Psychological Bulletin,* 117:387–403.

Van Ilzendoorn, M.H. & Kroonenberg, P.M. (1988). Cross-cultural patterns of attachment: A meta-analysis of the Strange Situation. *Child Development, 59,* 147–156.

Ventura, S.J., Martin, J.A., Mathews, T.J. & Clarke, S.C. (1996). Advance report of final natality statistics, 1994. *Monthly Vital Statistics Report, 44*(11), suppl. Hyattsville, MD: National Center for Health Statistics.

Ventura, S.J., Taffel, S.M., Mosher, W.D. Wilson, J.B. & Henshaw, S. (1995). Trends in pregnancies and pregnancy rates: Estimates for the United States, 1980–1992. *Monthly Vital Statistics Report, 43*(11), suppl. Hyattsville, MD: National Center for Health Statistics.

Vernon, M., Green, J. & Frothingham, T. (1983). Teenage pregnancy: A prospective study of self-esteem and other sociodemographic factors. *Pediatrics, 72,* 632–635.

Vygotsky, L. (1978). *Mind and society.* Cambridge MA: Harvard University Press.

Vygotsky, L.S. (1987). Thinking and speech. In R.W. Rieber & A.S. Carton (Eds.), *The collected works of L.S. Vygotsky. Vol. I: Problems of general psychology* (N. Minck, Trans.). New York: Plenum. (Original work published 1934.)

Walters, L.H., Walters, J. & McHenry, P. (1986). Differentiation of girls at risk of early pregnancy from the general population of adolescents. *Journal of Genetic Psychology, 148*(1), 19–29.

Ward, M.C. (1991, November). *The case of early childbearing: Where programs, policy and pregnancy intersect.* Paper presented at Wenner-Genn conference on politics of reproduction, Teresopolis, Brazil.

Ward, M.C. (1971). *Them children: A study in language learning.* New York: Holt, Rinehart & Winston.

Ward, M.J. & Carlson, E. (1991). *The predictive validity of the Adult Attachment*

Interview for adolescent mothers. Paper presented at the 59th meeting of the Society for Research in Child Development, Seattle, WA.

Ward, M.J. & Carlson, E. (1995). The predictive validity of the adult attachment interview for adolescent mothers. *Child Development, 66,* 69–79.

Washington, A.C. (1982). A cultural and historical prospective in pregnancy activity among U.S. teenagers. *Journal of Black Psychology, 9*(1), 1–28.

Waters, E., Crowell, J., Treboux, D., O'Connor, E. Posada, G., & Golby, B. (1993, April). *Discriminant validity of the Adult Attachment Interview.* Poster presented at the 60th meeting of the Society for Research in Child Development, New Orleans.

Watson, M.W. & Getz, K. (1990). Developmental shifts in oedipal behaviors related to family role understanding. In I. Bretherton & M.W. Watson (Eds.), *Children's perspectives on the family.* San Francisco: Jossey-Bass.

Williams, C. W. (1991). *Black teenage mothers.* Lexington, MA: Lexington Books.

Wilson, W.J. (1987). *The truly disadvantaged: The inner city, the underclass, and public policy.* Chicago: University of Chicago Press.

Wilson, W. J. & Neckerman, K. (1986). Poverty and family structure: The widening gap between evidence and public policy issues. In S. Danzier & D. Weinberg (Eds.), *Fighting poverty* (pp. 232–259). Cambridge, MA: Harvard University Press.

Young, V. H. (1970). Family and childhood in a southern Negro community. *American Anthropologist, 72,* 269–288.

Zongker, C.E. (1977). The self-concept of pregnant adolescent girls. *Adolescence, 12*(48), 477–488.

Index

B
Baird, A., 16, 59, 213, 232
Bakersmans-Kranenburg, J. J., 53n, 227
Barglow, P., 9, 18, 170, 227
Bates, E., 42, 227
Behavior
  adolescent pregnancy, 19
  multiple motivational sources of, 3
  sources of, ix, xii
Behavior pattern, adolescent pregnancy, 183, 184, 197
  intervention aimed at, 198
  perpetuation of, 42
Behavioral solution, adolescent pregnancy as problem and, 197
"Being on the make," 125
Belsky, J., 201, 227
Benigni, L., 42, 227
Benoit, D., 53n, 123, 227
Bernard, J., 23, 24, 227
"Best fit" model, 84n
Bibring, G. L., 9, 227
Bidell, T., 147, 184, 227
Bierman, B., 18, 170, 227
Bierman, J., 18, 170, 227
Billingsley, A., 21, 22, 227
Birth control, 71
  availability of, 3, 8
  knowledge, attitudes and beliefs about, 214–215
  mother's beliefs about, 81
  mother's not telling daughter about in inconsistent restrictive but noninformative schema, 68
  mother's willingness to give information on in inconsistent informative but nonrestrictive schema, 71–72
Birth control pills
  mothers' discouragement of daughters' use of, 66, 82, 88, 198
    in consistent nonrestrictive and noninformative schema, 77–78, 79

in inconsistent informative but nonrestrictive schema, 70, 71
in inconsistent restrictive but noninformative schema, 69
mother's putting daughter on, in consistent restrictive and informative schema, 74–75
Birth rates
  to adolescent girls, decline in, 197–198
  to unmarried teenagers, 6, 6n, 7f
    African American, 6, 6n, 7f, 187t
    white, 6, 6n, 7f, 187t
Biting reflex, 128
"Blame-the-victim" viewpoint, viii, 10, 90
Blassingame, J., 22, 23, 228
Blehar, M. C., 53, 141, 227
Blos, P., 9, 159n, 163n, 170, 228
  description of two types of female delinquents, 159n, 163
"Blue stone," 2
Bodily zones, 127
Bowlby, J., 12, 13, 54, 98, 138, 139, 140, 170, 228
  attachment theory, 138–140
  revised version of, 140
Breast, mother's withdrawal of, 128
Bretherton, I., 12, 13, 42, 54, 98, 122, 140, 141, 143, 144, 168, 170, 227, 228
Brody, 219
Brooks-Gunn, J., 9, 17, 196, 228, 230
Buchholz, E. S., 18, 170, 228
Burton, L. M., 18, 63, 228

C
Camaioni, L., 42, 227
Cannot classify category on AAI, 53, 56
Caregiver, *See also* Father; Mother; Parent
  functions of, 13
  insufficient feedback to child's signals, 144
  permitting of access to infant, 140